"The Successful Body *is ama_____ nary! This book is the gate that ____ ___ ____ ____ __ _____ ___ ___* ent visions and methods from highly skilled professionals on how to reach the peak of body functioning. The Successful Body *is not only a precious mine of information; it is a powerful motivator that will contribute to improving our lives.*"

—ALESSANDRO FIORENTINI,
CEO of Top Personal Trainers

"*Being truly healthy is a multi-faceted journey that takes a lot of work. The Successful Body addresses easy practical approaches one can use to weave fitness, nutrition, and mindset equally to live a healthier and happier life.*"

—Dr. STEM SITHEMBILE MAHLATINI,
Founder of The Empowerment Academy

"*If you are like me, you want to live as long and healthy a life as possible. Fortunately, Erik Seversen has put together an indispensable resource to live longer and better, compiling expert insight from some of the top minds in health and wellness. Whether you want to maximize your workouts, dial in your nutrition, or cultivate a stronger mindset, there is something in* The Successful Body *for you.*"

–ANDREW MERLE, Certified Sports Nutritionist,
Food & Health Writer

"The Successful Body *encompasses all aspects of health, including nutrition, physical activity and mental wellbeing, needed to create life changing, sustainable habits. These 33 global experts not only share their own personal stories as they relate to their field of expertise, but also provide practical pointers to motivate and help readers!*"

—SERRA TUMAY, MS, RD;
Founder of Tohum Nutrition

"Wellness is determined by choices people make in how to live their lives. To have an optimal quality of life is dependent on nutrition, fitness, and mindset. The Successful Body *is a collection of knowledge by professionals from all over the world. This collective effort provides the information necessary to start on the path to creating wellness in one's life. From ancient techniques to cutting edge ideas, this book is a great place to start."*

—BRIAN XICOTENCATL, Founder of Water Polo Strong, Co-Owner of Breathe Performance

"The Successful Body *gives you the answers you need to have a healthy life. By reading this book, you will find clues on how to get in shape and deal with stress. You will learn to evoke a positive mentality and know the benefits of making healthy choices while taking control of your negative thoughts, so they don't affect your physical well-being. I believe Erik Seversen found the best experts to represent in his book."*

—BEN CHRISTIAN, Certified Personal Trainer, Inspirational Writer

"Do you know that your body knows everything? We often overlook our body wisdom even though the secret to success may lie in the trinity of a healthy body, healthy mind, and healthy spirit. This book provides you with wisdom, knowledge, and practical tips to gain your body wisdom from 33 global body experts offering diverse perspectives on various body topics. The Successful Body *is the perfect companion to Erik Seversen's previous book,* The Successful Mind, *written by 33 global mindset experts. I refer to these brilliant books as my precious resource library on all things body and mind."*

—RÚNA BOUIUS, Founder of True Power Institute and author of *Burnout Busters*

THE
SUCCESSFUL
BODY

THE SUCCESSFUL BODY

Using Fitness, Nutrition, and Mindset to Live Better

Authored by:

Erik Seversen, Nancy Addison, Sébastien Assohou, Arianna Auñón, Marian Bourne, Kyle Coletti, Toni Delos Santos, Laura Eiman, Patricia Faust, Chelsea Fournier, Rolando Garcia III, Roy E. Hatcher, Sarah Jones, Shira Litwack, Dee McKee, Shane McShea, Jenna Minecci, Selena Ella Moon, Kealah Parkinson, Robert Prokop, Wendy Quan, Jay Quarmby, James Rizzo, Jeannette Ruiz, Christina Santini, Paul Scianna, Rocky Snyder, Johnny Spilotro, Denise E. Stegall, Vince Stevenson, Fozi Stinson, Leslie M. Thornton, David H. Wallis, M.D., Dave White, PhD

THIN LEAF PRESS | LOS ANGELES

Library of Congress Cataloging-in-Publication Data
Names: Seversen, Erik, Author, et al.

Title: The Successful Body: Using Fitness, Nutrition, and Mindset to Live Better

LCCN 2020924669
ISBN 978-1-953183-00-2 | ISBN 978-1-953183-01-9 (ebook)
Nonfiction, Health, Fitness, Nutrition, Mind, Body & Spirit
Cover Design: 100 Covers
Interior Design: Formatted Books
Editor: Nancy Pile
Copy Editor: Rebecca Lau
Thin Leaf Press
Los Angeles

THIN
LEAF

Thank you for reading this book. There are tools found within the following pages that can greatly benefit your life, but don't stop there. Make sure you get the most you can from this book and reach out directly to the 33 expert authors who want to help you enjoy life with a healthy body and fit mind. Contact information for each author is found at the end of their respective chapter.

To the coaches, trainers, and doctors, who transform people's lives daily, and to those who are ready to make positive transformations in their own lives.

CONTENTS

INTRODUCTION

By Erik Seversen
Author of *Ordinary to Extraordinary* and *Explore*
Los Angeles, California

As I completed my book *Explore*, I was anxious to get another book written about happiness and success. I gathered the help of 33 world-class experts to co-write the book, *The Successful Mind*. This book was a massive success. It became a bestseller in the USA and the United Kingdom and remained a bestseller for weeks. On top of that, the Ministry of Culture in Syria asked if they could look into having the book translated into Arabic to reach a wider audience. What I like best about *The Successful Mind* is that I've received countless thanks and feedback from regular individuals, ranging from struggling students to high-powered executives, about how something in the book sparked a positive change in their lives. I decided I didn't want the influence of these positive changes to stop there. And so, the idea of producing a related book—*The Successful Body*—was created.

As with *The Successful Mind*, I began reaching out to a variety of experts who could contribute something unique to the book, and I intentionally looked for individuals who are extremely successful in their fields, who come from a variety of different backgrounds, and who work in diverse areas of expertise. My goal was not to have a group of authors with the same opinion about the body, health, and success, but rather to have multiple perspectives. As a result, *The Successful Body* was created by a group of 33 top experts in health and wellness, who each help answer the question: *what is the most important thing a person can do to create more success in their business and their life by using fitness, nutrition, and mindset?*

In this book, you'll encounter the answer to this question from 33 experts from a variety of backgrounds. These contributors come from all over the USA, all over Canada, the United Kingdom, Ireland, Denmark, France, Spain, and Australia. These authors' areas of expertise include stress management, treatment of chronic illness, sports psychology, gerontology, brain health, mental toughness, neuroscience, wellness, biohacking, nutrigenomics, fitness, kettlebells, yoga, Pilates, strength conditioning, injury rehabilitation, fight-or-flight stress response, corporate mindfulness, meditation, nutrition, CrossFit, transformational therapy, biological medicine, medical thermography, environmental toxins, neurolinguistic programming, hypnotherapy, chronic inflammation, oxidative stress, holistic health and nutrition, addiction recovery, kinesiology, pain management, sports medicine, and more.

The authors composing this book are medical doctors, nurses, PhDs, multiple bestselling authors, international keynote speakers, workshop facilitators, gym and fitness center owners, military soldiers, podcast hosts, radio show hosts, CEOs and founders of health-related companies, professional athletes, martial arts experts, gold medal Olympic weightlifting champions, body builders, fitness instructors, personal trainers, Ironman triathletes, marathoners, NCAA referees, chefs, scientists, and nutritionists.

The authors composing this book have been featured on NBC, Fox, CBS, Spike TV, National French, Italian, Spanish, Australian, and Chinese television and radio programs, *Forbes*, *New York Post*, and many more internationally recognized media outlets. They have worked in health-industry businesses, including Golds Gym, Powerhouse Gym, Retro Fitness, Tapout Fitness, Equinox, Orangetheory, and many more. Also, these authors have received honors including "Athlete of the Year" from the US Olympic Committee, praise such as "America's Next Fitness Phenomenon," recognition for research from University of California, Berkeley, and endorsements from individuals, including Oprah, Rachel Ray, and Barbara Walters. In summary, the individuals who contributed to this book are people who have gone beyond the normal levels of fitness and nutrition and are health-industry leaders who all want to help you find the best you possible.

The Successful Body is divided into three areas: fitness, nutrition, and mindset. These are three easily identifiable "parts" of success that can be measured as they transform in your life. You can witness tangible transformations in weight, tone, energy alertness, and mental outlook. Each chapter highlights one of the three aspects—fitness, nutrition, or mindset—as its main focus, but as most authors work with a holistic approach, almost every chapter speaks toward all three of these, even if the main idea of the chapter focuses on one.

Although this book is organized around the united theme of health and personal growth, each chapter is totally stand-alone. The chapters in this book can be read in any order. I encourage you to look through the table of contents and begin wherever you want. Even still, I urge you to read all the chapters because, as a whole, they provide a great array of perspectives with each one proving valuable in providing you tools for the creation of a successful body.

While I'm extremely proud of the information contained within the chapters in this book, nothing can replace the real communication and accountability offered through face-to-face or online instruction. If you connect with something within this book, I encourage you to reach out to the author directly. Each of them wants to help you live the best, most healthy, satisfied life you can. I pray that this book is instrumental in helping you feel better, look better, and reach your goals.

Email: Erik@ErikSeversen.com
Website: www.ErikSeversen.com

CHAPTER 1

FUNDAMENTALS OF HEALTHY EATING

By Nancy Addison CHC, AADP
Founder of Organic Healthy Lifestyle
Dallas, Texas

Take care of your body. It's the only place you have to live.
—Jim Rohn

We all want to be our healthiest and have radiance from the inside out—so where do we start? The following words act as a no-nonsense list of things you can do right away to improve your body—and life—through the foods you eat. While I've written volumes about health, nutrition, and cooking, below are some of my top tips for obtaining a healthier life and lifestyle. While I don't particularly like "do and don't" lists, sometimes the easiest way to see exactly where to start is by just such assertions, so for these very fundamental aspects of nutrition, let's just get to it.

1. **Eat high-quality, nutrient-dense foods.** Our well-being depends on the quality of our food.
2. **Eat organic and non-GMO foods.** Because what we eat becomes our blood, tissues, and cells, I recommend buying organic whenever possible. If we eat foods that either have toxic herbicides sprayed on

them or have been altered by genetically modifying their seeds to have had poisons placed into them, then we ingest poison.

3. **Avoid processed foods.** Choose unprocessed foods, so you aren't ingesting MSG, potassium bromate, aspartame, wood pulp, artificial dyes, chemicals, and other additives that are put in processed food.

4. **Eat more raw whole foods.** Eating organic, live, fresh, vine-ripened or tree-ripened whole food can feed the body on a deeper cellular level than cooked or processed foods. Vine- or tree-ripened foods have salvestrols in them that have cancer-fighting properties.

5. **Eat a varied diet.** Keep a variety of seasonal fresh fruits and vegetables in your diet.

6. **Eat whole sprouted seeds and grains.** When eating pasta, bread, crackers, and chips, consume only whole sprouted grains. Avoid corn and wheat, especially non-organic and genetically modified varieties. Gluten-free and sprouted grains are preferable.

7. **Cut out sugar or consume as little as possible.** Do not use fake sugar substitutes in any way, shape, or form. Avoid any kind of high fructose sugar added to foods, like high fructose corn syrup or agave nectar. My recommended choices for healthier sweeteners are date sugar and raw organic honey.

8. **Eat plant-based, high-protein, and nutrient-rich foods daily.** Make sure you are not low in any nutrients. Consume whole, sprouted, organic, cooked lentils, quinoa, beans, and legumes regularly for the complex amino acids that are the building blocks of protein. Ensure that all the B vitamins, especially B12, are in your diet and absorbed well. Iodine, iron, zinc, vitamin D, vitamin C, sulfur, chromium, magnesium, selenium, minerals, and complex amino acids are all important nutrients and should not be overlooked.

9. **Consume only good fats like organic extra virgin coconut oil or olive oil.** Make sure you get enough of the essential fatty acids— omega-3, in particular.

10. **Chew food thoroughly to aid digestion.** Avoid drinking beverages with your meals. Beverages water down the digestive juices, making them less acidic. This makes it harder for the body to digest food.

Hydration Is Paramount!

Now, let's move on to hydration. Water is a key ingredient to our health and well-being because, according to Medical News Today, our body's composition averages 60 percent water with the range going as high as 75 percent water. In our body, teeth have the least amount of water at 8 to 10 percent, and the kidneys and the brain contain the most water at 80 to 85 percent. Doesn't that make you want to pay attention to how much water you get?

Blood, which is 50 percent water, uses water to transport oxygen, nutrients, and antibodies to all parts of the body. Many illnesses are actually a result of dehydration, so it is important to maintain an adequate intake of water throughout the day. By the time you feel thirsty, you are already dehydrated.

Some good hydrating fluids include not only regular, plain water, but also other drinks that give you water, such as tea, vegetable and fruit juices, milks (including non-dairy milks), broths/soups, and coconut water. You also get water from the food you eat. An average food provides about 20 percent of your total fluid intake.

When you choose your hydrating fluids, it is important to be aware that in addition to containing water, they can also provide essential vitamins and minerals that give you energy and nutrition as well.

Ready for a few more "dos and don'ts"? Some main components for keeping optimum hydration are:

1. Drink a sufficient amount of water (or hydrating fluid). **Drink an ounce of water for every two pounds of body weight daily.** This means that someone weighing 200 pounds should drink 100 ounces of water a day. This is in addition to any other beverages. For best results, consume water the first thing upon getting up in the morning, and then drink it all day long on a continual basis every two hours, as long as you avoid having it with meals or snacks.
2. **Avoid drinking water (or liquids) with meals.** As already mentioned, doing this can dilute the digestive enzyme juices, making it harder to digest food. It is best to drink water between meals, not during meals. Drink water two hours after a meal or one hour before a meal.
3. **Drink and bathe in water that is pure and free of chlorine and fluoride.** Be mindful of the source of the water you drink, bathe, and swim in. Almost all public water supplies have chemicals added, including sodium fluoride and chlorine, both of which are poisons.

The two main chemicals added to water supplies include chlorine and fluoride.

Chlorine was the first poison developed for warfare. It destroys vitamin E in the body and the good probiotics in the intestines. According to Emily Sohn on NBC News, Industrial chemist J.P. Bercz, PhD, showed in 1992 that chlorinated water alters and destroys unsaturated essential fatty acids (EFAs), the building blocks of people's brains and central nervous systems.

Fluoride is a cumulative poison. On average, only 50 percent of the fluoride we ingest each day is excreted through the kidneys. The remainder accumulates in our bones, pineal gland, and other tissues. If the kidney is damaged, fluoride accumulation will increase, and with it, the likelihood of harm. Fluoride affects the thyroid gland, and all our enzymatic systems. Side effects from fluoride ingestion include weight problems, damage to our immune system, and other serious disorders. The effects of fluoride vary from person to person, and these affects even. vary depending on a person's age.

To Salt or Not to Salt

When I ask people if they use salt, they frequently tell me, "No, I eat a low-salt diet for health reasons." In fact, it is not salt that is bad for us, it is the *type* of salt we eat.

The word "electrolyte" is a chemical term for salt. We need electrolytes to be healthy. As thyroid expert Dr. David Brownstein says, "Without salt, life itself would not be possible." The misconception about salt stems from the fact that conventional medical doctors make no differentiation between white, refined salt and unrefined, mineral-rich sea salt.

Unrefined sea salt is important for life because it promotes the proper balance for the endocrine, adrenal, and thyroid glands to function properly; supports healthy blood pressure; detoxifies the body; and, along with water, is necessary for the optimal functioning of the immune system, hormonal system, and cardiovascular health.

Sea salt can also help balance the body by alkalizing it. Maintaining a slightly alkaline pH is important to our health.

The white, refined table salt that most of us grew up using lacks numerous minerals that are present in whole, unrefined salt. Refined table salt is 98 percent sodium chloride with added bicarbonates, chemicals, sugar, and preservatives. Iodine, the main nutrient that supports our thyroid gland, is added to many refined salts, but in insufficient quantities to prevent thyroid illnesses and other iodine needs of the body. Given that iodine dissipates after being exposed to oxygen, table salt could never be a reliable source of iodine anyway.

Many food sources today lack vital minerals and nutrients. Soils are depleted, and refining and processing take out many or all the nutrients in foods. Salt cravings are actually a signal you may be depleted in nutrients, minerals, and electrolytes.

Dr. David Brownstein says low-salt diets "promote toxicity" and have adverse effects on numerous metabolic markers, including promoting elevated insulin levels and insulin resistance. Low-salt diets have been associated with elevating normal cholesterol and LDL cholesterol levels, which, in turn, have been associated with cardiovascular disease. Finally, low-salt diets will lead to mineral deficiencies and the development of chronic disease.

In 1994, The *British Medical Journal* published a study conducted in the Netherlands. In this study, common refined table salt was replaced with mineral salt that was naturally high in magnesium and potassium. Half of the group was taken off of their high blood pressure medication and put on an unrefined, mineral-rich salt ingredient diet. Notice that they simply changed this one *type* of food—salt—in their diet. This group showed a reduction in blood pressure equivalent to that produced by the blood pressure-lowering pharmaceutical drugs.

Healthy Fats

Healthy fats are essential for our overall health and well-being. Healthy fats are raw, unprocessed, organic fats in their natural form. The advertising industry would have us believe that all fat is bad or fattening. But actually, good fat can be critical to maintaining our health and controlling our weight. Fat tells the body how to utilize protein and carbohydrates. Fat can make our food taste richer and more satisfying, and good fats are vital for good brain health.

Trans fats, however, should be avoided completely. Trans fats are hydrogenated fats that have been chemically changed to stay solid at room temperature and have an extremely long shelf life, which is not their natural state. This type of fat is unhealthy, even in tiny amounts.

Essential Fatty Acids

Essential fatty acids, i.e., omega-3s, are called "essential" because they are not made by our body and must be obtained through the diet.

Because they have anti-inflammatory properties, omega-3s help with the prevention of many health problems: heart disease, rheumatoid arthritis, macular degeneration, asthma, eczema, other immune dysfunctions, and cancer. Omega-3s also help with improving memory and can help improve mood. A deficiency may appear as inflammation, water retention, and high blood pressure.

Make essential fatty acids a regular part of your diet, but always use fresh, cold-pressed oils and refrigerate them. This is crucial because essential fatty acids can become rancid and create free radicals in the body, which will foster aging and a weakened immune system.

Choose organic, whole-food, cold-pressed, unprocessed good fats and enjoy your food. Don't feel guilty about adding healthy fat to recipes. Your body and brain will be glad you did!

Types of Healthy Fats/Oils

Coconut oil, a type of "nut" fat, is highly effective as an antioxidant. In most parts of the world, it is seen as the superfood of fats. It is a unique saturated fat and a medium-chain fatty acid, which means that pancreatic enzymes or bile are not required for the body to process it. This also means it is easily absorbed by the body. Coconut oil nourishes the body, and the medium-chain fatty acids provide a good source of energy. Also, the lauric acid in coconut oil is a natural immune system booster. For years, many people thought coconut oil was bad for your health because it raised cholesterol. But in actuality, it provides good cholesterol (HDL).

Pure coconut oil has many benefits, including:

- promoting heart health
- supporting immune system health
- supporting a healthy metabolism
- providing an immediate energy source
- helping to keep skin healthy and youthful looking
- supporting the proper functioning of the thyroid gland

Olive oil is a wonderful, unique ingredient. It is an omega-9, monounsaturated, long-chain fatty acid, and is the only vegetable oil that can be pressed and used in its pure form. The key ingredient found in olive oil is oleic acid. Extra virgin olive oil has more vitamin E in it than other types of olive oil.

Olive oil can become rancid if heated or stored improperly. It needs to be kept refrigerated and away from light. It should be used only with recipes and food preparation that don't require it to be heated, unless it says on the label it is meant to handle high heat.

Hemp oil contains significant amounts of omega-3s and omega-6s. Hemp oil also contains significant amounts of Vitamin E, which is important for the thyroid gland.

Flax seeds are one of the best sources of omega-3 essential fatty acids. They are rich in alpha-linolenic acid, fiber, and lignans. Lignans are phytoestrogens, or plant compounds that have an estrogen-like effect, with antioxidant properties. These lignans can help stabilize hormone levels and reduce PMS and menopause symptoms.

Alpha-linolenic acid is anti-inflammatory. It promotes the lowering of C-reactive protein in the blood, which is a biomarker of inflammation.

Chia seeds have more omega-3 fatty acids than Atlantic salmon. But, unlike salmon, chia seeds are about 10 percent omega-6 oil. They are a more perfect balance of omega fats, with a ratio of three omega-3s to one omega-6. Along with the rich omega oils, chia seeds have almost five times more calcium than milk; one ounce of chia has 179 mg calcium, and one ounce of whole milk has 36 mg calcium; more antioxidants than fresh blueberries; and more protein, calcium, and fiber than flax seeds. Chia seeds are one of the best nutrient-dense superfoods around.

So, from eating more chemical-free, unadulterated foods, drinking the correct amount of water, and managing sugar, salt, fats, and oils, you can transform your life by making relatively simple changes to your diet. If you are looking for a quick transformation in your health, study all the details in the above suggestions and begin a regimen of eating better. Or, just select even one or two things to start with and gradually build as you improve your eating and your health. Either way, you will improve the successful functioning of your body. The important thing is just to become aware of what you're putting into your body and decide what type of outcomes you'd like to enjoy.

About the Author

Nancy Gibbons Addison CHC, AADP shatters the stereotype about healthy eating. This unique nutritionist cuts through the myths and misinformation about health and nutrition. If you want the straight and honest truth, with easy ways to take control of your health and reverse disease, you want to ask Nancy.

Nancy is a bestselling and award-winning author, an international speaker, radio and podcast show host, chef, and counselor. Offering much more than a "diet," Nancy's speeches, radio shows, six books, and numerous articles offer a constantly expanding body of knowledge that focuses on the benefits of establishing and maintaining a healthy body, mind, and spirit. She has also appeared on NBC, Fox, CBS, BronxNet, etc., and in documentaries, including *Eating You Alive*. You can reach Nancy on her website, Organic Healthy Life, or find easy, healthy recipes in Nancy's nutrition-packed books, which are half-cookbooks, on Nancy's author page.

Email: nancy@nancyaddison.com
Website: www.organichealthylife.com
Author Page: https://www.amazon.com/Nancy-Addison/e/B00E6K5KGY/

CHAPTER 2
SELF-KNOWLEDGE AND CARING

By Sébastien Assohou
Life Coach, Personal Trainer, Entrepreneur
Paris, France

Anxiety is a thin stream of fear trickling through the mind. If encouraged,
it cuts a channel into which all other thoughts are drained.
—Somers Roche

I am fascinated by cognitive neurosciences and biomechanics, and I've always been compelled to share with others about the needs and workings of the majestic machine that is the human body.

My attraction to neuroscience and biomechanics is most certainly related to my professions, first, as an athlete, and second, as a police officer with the French government. My experiences both as an athlete and police officer trained me to push myself beyond my limits to the highest performance of body and mind. Furthermore, as a life coach, I strive to raise awareness among my clients on how to nourish their bodies.

Something I commonly say is, "Our greatest wealth is to be able to feed our brain with knowledge, so invest in yourself," and I have witnessed extremely positive results from people who choose to invest in their own bodies and minds. I'm happy you are choosing to invest in yourself right now.

The human body contains functioning elements that are not visible from the naked eye, such as cells and globules. The human body requires the combination of the following three elements to achieve stability and balance, both physically and mentally: physical activity, psychological well-being, and a healthy, balanced diet. British botanist Arthur George Tansley, who coined the term "ecosystem," analyzed "complex organisms and physical factors," with a "physical factor" referring to that in the abiotic environment that influences the growth and development of organisms of biological communities. This bond between complex organisms and physical factors is constantly evolving. There also must be a perfect symbiosis between the three elements of physical activity, psychological well-being, and healthy diet to take full advantage of their benefits.

In my work as a life coach, I emphasize the importance of this symbiosis of mental health, physical health, and nutrition to create what is called "homeostasis," which is the maintenance of the regulation of the internal constants of the body, such as body temperature, heart rate, respiratory functions, or the circulation of fluids and gases, at a stable level.

The main enemy of our ecosystem and, according to US National Institute of Health, the number one killer in the USA is **stress**, which is defined as negative emotional and physical tension in the body. The stress reaction can lead to digestive disorders, headaches, sleep disturbances, but also other physiological disorders, such as diabetes, obesity, cardiovascular problems, strokes, and many other serious conditions.

Stress, however, is not always negative. The training I received taught me to turn stress into positive energy. It is important to face stress head-on, and this intention comes from our brain. The brain and the body are two very distinct entities whose common function is to maintain our physical and mental state in perfect connection to optimize our body's protection system. If stress is pervasive, depending on an individual's particular personality traits, the brain can integrate it into habits or even become chronic.

I've already mentioned the importance of the balance of exercise, well-being, and diet. Now, let me reveal how you can use these to fight stress and even to turn stress into strength.

Physical Activity

Let's start with the importance of physical activity. One of our societal problems is that many people focus solely on the physical appearance, especially with the increase of social networks and advertisements that highlight certain types of physical beauty. People always feel the pressure of being physically judged. This is presumably why many of my new client's goals are simply to transform their bodies. But during our sessions, their body transformation results in inner confidence.

If you want to take ownership of your life, I recommend integrating physical exercise into your daily routine. Daily exercise can take the form of daily tasks such as taking the stairs instead of the elevator, riding a bicycle instead of using public transportation, making phone calls while walking, and so on. Carrying out these types of physical activities strengthens the immune system, increases the metabolism, oxygenates the brain, and makes the brain more efficient. I voluntarily choose not to use the word "sport" but to use the term "physical activity" because even one hour of any activity per day is enough to keep the body in shape. If you commit to this day after day, you will gain confidence and self-esteem, which, in turn, decreases your stress levels.

At 14 years of age, when I started competing in sports, my stress was linked to the desire to do well and the desire to win. I had the choice to either let myself be overwhelmed by this stress or to face it. One of the techniques I used, and still use today, is deep, slow breathing because it activates the diaphragm and allows the control of the heart rate, thereby lowering the heart rate considerably. Deep, slow breathing creates endurance, and deep, slow breathing is very good for you, especially when you are sitting for long periods.

Here is an exercise you can try at home. Sit with your back straight and shut your eyes. Visualize a place that is comfortable and restful; focus on the quality and frequency of your breathing, which should be deep and slow, and try to think of positive and comforting thoughts. Breathe in through your nose by sucking air into your stomach and letting your lungs soak up the air; then, hold your breathing for a few seconds before exhaling very slowly through your mouth until all the air in your lungs is expelled.

When we control our breathing through mediation or physical activity, both the heart-rate and stress levels decrease. So, we can see that both sports and the simple act of breathing deeply can positively affect both the body and the brain.

Psychological Well-Being

It is important to condition the brain to gradually take over your emotional state. To be able to do this will allow you to value yourself and to gain confidence. More confidence translates to less stress. To do this, you must get out of your comfort zone to challenge your limits in order to achieve rewards on both physiological and psychological levels. I recommend doing a sport activity daily to promote neuromuscular exchanges and to release hormones, particularly oxytocin, also known as the "confidence hormone."

The brain is the seat of cognitive functions and sends electrical impulses to our organs and muscles. It has a connection throughout our body and coordinates our actions and keeps our vital organs operational. The brain is said to be plastic, meaning easily molded, which means that it is constantly evolving throughout our lives. It weighs less than 4.4 pounds and uses more than 20 percent of our daily energy. It is no wonder that the brain favors habits or the conditioning of our actions because that requires less energy.

During my duties as a police officer, our training was essentially based on learning new movements by repetition to be memorized by our brains. Consistent repetition of 300 or 400 times strengthens brain circuits and eventually makes them permanent. Two hours of repetitive exercises will be enough to create new synapses, which, in turn, encourages your brain to function more fully versus getting stuck in a circle of habits.

If we want to optimize brain function, we must act with willpower. The desire to improve is not enough, we must have the intention to undertake and put things into action. The goal of the exercises during training was to maintain the appropriate technical gestures without allowing ourselves to be disturbed by an emotional state that would jeopardize the mission. Studies observing the brain reveal that the hypertrophy area of the hippocampus thickens with experience and regresses when not perpetually stimulated, which is why doing the exercises repeatedly over two hours creates results.

Healthy, Balanced Diet

Let me tell you now of the importance of nutrition within the ecosystem.

As a life coach, the successful results of my clients depend greatly on their nutrition. The benefits of physical or intellectual activity are in equal importance to caloric and energetic intake to your body. Nutrition plays a vital role in the development of your cells and the proper functioning of your complex organism. Nutrients—proteins, lipids, and carbohydrates—are molecules produced during the digestion of the food we eat. These three groups allow your body to build itself, to renew itself, and to provide the energy necessary for your metabolism. Food and water are the body's fuel. By hydrating regularly, the body promotes the connection between your brain and body. This is why it is essential to respect a balanced diet by eating healthy foods with as little processing as possible.

Nutrients can be divided into two groups: essential nutrients and non-essential nutrients. Proteins and lipids are said to be essential because our body is unable to manufacture them; therefore, they must be provided through food, unlike carbohydrates, which can be synthesized from other nutrients.

Stress does not come only from external events. Diet is a contributing factor. Eating saturated fatty foods, foods rich in saturated carbohydrates, or overeating, forces the body to protect itself. These can trigger stress in the body when it carries out a chemical reaction, such as bloating, for example. But, through selecting health foods in the right amount, we can avoid this.

While performing duties for my police guard and protection unit, I often ate in the car with my partner because of a lack of time. We would compare our meals; mine were well-prepared, balanced meals, and his were often nutrition-low sandwiches purchased from a bakery or processed, ready-made meals from the grocery store. As a result, my partner often had stomachaches or fatigue, simply due to the work that his body had to go through while struggling with this junk food during digestion and neutralizing its absorption in an attempt to avoid polluting the body. When you eat a standard grocery store sandwich, you swallow chemical products because these sandwiches are made from unhealthy, addictive products. Typically, grocery store sandwiches are mainly made of sugar, salt, and taste enhancers, which are very bad for the body, versus homemade sandwiches in which you know all the ingredients. That's why I highly recommend preparing your own meals as much as possible, or at least, attempt to buy foods with unprocessed products.

Through my experiences, I have been made aware of the importance of the ecosystem, so I have come up with an easy way to remember this. I call it the "MPC Vision." I use this daily, both for myself and with my clients, as a way of providing the necessary weapons to face the difficulties of everyday-life health risks. In MPC, the M is for motivation, the P is for perseverance, and the C is for confidence.

- **Motivation (emotion).** Whether social, sentimental, or professional, motivation is the key to your success. It is the driving force behind your actions.

- **Perseverance (reasoning).** Perseverance is a major asset in achieving your goal. It can be related to the fuel that powers your engine. Motivation and perseverance are, therefore, closely linked.
- **Confidence (factual).** Without confidence and trust, you will allow yourself to be overwhelmed and destabilized by the judgment of the outside world. Confidence and trust would have the same function as a shield that protects you from the influence of others.

The MPC Vision is my simple reminder to encourage you to take charge of yourself and to find and maintain your right balance of exercise, well-being, and eating habits. If you maintain this action over time, the positive effects will work on your body and your mind. You will become aware that you are capable of taking charge of your body, so you can become the best version of yourself.

About the Author

Sébastien Assohou, simply nicknamed "Badoun" by his friends and clients, is a personal trainer and life coach. He supervises a portfolio of selected clients worldwide and shares his expertise on sports, health, and well-being through various French media, including television, radio, magazines, and online. Sébastien works with executives, high-performance clients, and those seeking to make a significant, permanent, and healthier life change.

Sébastien's experience, which covers special forces training, presidential security, professional sports, fitness education, nutrition consulting, life coaching, and business management, brings a unique perspective to the world of coaching and fitness. His approach is based on the belief that all people are multidimensional. Health and fitness are closely linked to your mental health, your performance at work, and even your relationships. By considering each client as a whole person, he has helped clients find an uncommon degree of success in achieving real and positive change.

Email: contact@sebastienassohou.com
LinkedIn: https://www.linkedin.com/in/sebastien-assohou/

CHAPTER 3

LIBERATE YOUR BODY THROUGH CELLULAR NUTRITION

By Arianna Auñón
Nutritionist, Women's Health Specialist and Mentor
Ibiza, Spain

What you seek is seeking you.
—Rumi

We are led to believe that the more vitamins, the more minerals, the more protein, and the more good fats we eat, the healthier we'll be. This is a lie.

What changed everything for me when it came to transforming my body, my mind, and even my fitness was learning that truly embodying health entailed cleaning my body at a cellular level with foods that actually heal, cleanse, and regenerate the body, not further clogging it up with too much high fat, protein, and toxins. This process I created was like finding a cave full of precious diamonds that so few know about. It taught me a way of standing like a lioness, out of the box, out of the mainstream, and doing things differently. I realised what I had to do to embody ultimate health and the truth in my body. This, I found out, is total and utter BLISS, JOY, FREEDOM, and HAPPINESS. This place can be a permanent heaven-on-earth that starts inside you. It is available for everyone. No one is lucky. Those who get the incredible results are the ones who commit, who decide, who have a big WHY, who don't settle for just okay-good-fine, but GO for their wildest dreams and vision. YOU have that potential right now.

When I decided to commit to a new way, an evolved way, a deeply conscious way of BEing in my body, divine steps unfolded … I listened and absorbed breadcrumbs that were guiding me home. So, if you are reading this, YAY! I am so happy you have your hands on this very sacred process that transformed my physical, mental, emotional, and spiritual health completely. Through this process, I remembered my true self, my heart, a homecoming. Finally, I felt fully at home and at peace in my own body, as me.

Through the process I outline, you can also remember the love you are made of. Here you get to feel, hear, see, and know the TRUTH again, as you peel away all those layers of toxins, waste, mucus, parasites, stones, heavy metals, plaque, and all that gunk that lies deep in the body at a cellular level, keeping you from feeling your best. It is the chemicals, the acidic residue, that makes you feel awful, exhausted, heavy, foggy, anxious, stressed, lacking in confidence, gaining weight, hormonal, stuck, frustrated, and stagnant. All of this, of course, impacts the mind because your mind is in every cell of your being. Many toxins are stored in the liver, your biggest internal organ, and the liver is also connected to the mind. An inflamed, stressed liver is an inflamed, stressed mind.

The relationship we have with ourselves, with our body, is the relationship we have with everything else: food, other people, loved ones, money, life …
It's all a reflection of the relationship we have with our own body.

There is no disease, there is dis-ease, and dis-ease in the body only arises into physical symptoms when the body is obstructed with waste. You must remove the cellular acidic residue that is making you think you want acidic food. When your soul says no to acidic food and residue, a shift is made, and you remember your natural state of being liberated, healthy, and happy.

"So how do I get to this liberated state?" I can hear you asking. It all starts with "luxurious alkaline living", I like to call it. True luxury starts inside your own sacred body temple with what you feed it. Eating at least 80 percent alkaline, mucus-free, whole-plant foods, cleaning and detoxing as you effortlessly merge with your day-to-day life, is a process. It takes time to get to this point, and this is where we are going together. I'm going to show you how to create an alkaline life.

Did you know the human is an alkaline-dominant creature? We are YIN creatures, feminine, we come from nature. Why do you feel at such peace in nature? Because you are nature. Your true self is still, sacred, abundant, relaxed, peaceful, free. Your true self is flowing as nature. On the contrary, much of the conditioning around life is about being busy, doing to get, doing to feel enough. The conditioned belief that relaxing is lazy and being busy is important is what leads so many people to distraction, drama, and addiction.

*Nature reminds you of your true self … It's here, it's still, and
with it, you get to deepen into the arms of self-love.*

The transition into an alkaline life is a very sacred transition process. I will be sharing seven steps to integrate into your life. This process has given me so much freedom, peace, healing, confidence, joy, happiness, and optimal health. It has allowed me to remember my divinity and heal what most would say is incurable. *Anything is possible.*

I always feel fully supported, nourished, and healthy in my body when I stick to this method that I call *The Body Awakening*, and I remember that I AM a GodGoddess.

Before I dive into the seven-step process, I want to share something about nutrition since nutrition has been one of my greatest journeys ever.

Nutrition holds the FREEDOM you are seeking.

Where My Journey Started

I grew up in Devon, United Kingdom, in the beauty of the countryside, rolling green hills. My dad was a head chef for over 40 years, and my mum an incredible baker and cook too. Food was a big deal in our household. We were such foodies that as we were eating breakfast, we'd be talking about lunch, and when eating lunch, we'd be talking about dinner. This went on and on.

For me, food became very emotional, an attachment, escape, excuse, and addiction. I started to emotionally eat from a young age, not knowing then that's what was happening. This led me to an eating disorder, hormonal imbalance, severe anxiety, weight fluctuations, suppressed feelings, stress, a toxic gut, and an unclear mind. I also had an overburdened liver, kidneys, digestive system, and numbing in my body, and I was totally obstructed with acidic waste. This altered my internal environment to a state of dis-ease. I craved so many foods, mostly sweet, carby, fatty, creamy foods and drinks. At the time, I just wanted it, and I thought my body needed it. Maybe you can resonate with this?

Fast-forwarding to the present moment, I have learnt through studies and personal experience that the core to great health is cellular alkaline transitioning away from some of the quick-fix fad diets that once seemed so appealing to me.

I grew up eating it all—meat, eggs, fish, cow's milk, clotted cream, yoghurt, cakes, doughnuts, milk chocolate, croissants, and I was drinking a lot of alcohol, caffeine, and fizzy stuff. After all of this, I then went on to eat as a pescatarian and vegetarian. This wasn't for me, so I went back to eating everything. Going back to my old diet wasn't because I didn't like the foods I was eating. It was because my body was full of acidic residue, and it was the parasites I spoke about that were craving the foods for me. It wasn't me craving this acidic food; it was the stuff inside me causing the cravings. Then, I went on to veganism. I dropped in and out of veganism for a few years, felt good, felt terrible, and then decided I wanted to understand more about the food I was eating.

I decided I didn't want to eat animals any longer. I was feeling this real pull in my heart to stop, as it simply didn't feel good any more. It felt out of harmony with my body, which is part of our planet. I thought, "What we feed our body, we feed our planet family too".

I dived deep and found out how to eat vegan well. I felt good, but veganism still didn't give me the health freedom I was looking for. It was one of the many stepping stones I took until I landed on the rare diamond of the *cellular way* to health. I awoke one day, and everything shifted, and I started living 80 percent mucus-free because of *The Body Awakening* method that I created. Since then, I've shared this guide with my one-on-one clients and multiple retreat clients. Through this very process, they are set up for life-long health, and this is what I am going to share with you here. I think of this as next-level liberation. *The Body Awakening* method is a seven-step process to total health and freedom at every level of your being.

Of course, there will always be tweaks and tailoring because your journey is different from mine. We all store different experiences, emotions, traumas, toxicities, and memories deep in our cells. There are specific processes to go through to heal and unravel this, but I've seen the seven steps of *The Body*

Awakening method work with many individuals from different backgrounds. The seven steps are:

1. Nature's Natural Rhythms
2. Cellular Remove, Repair, Reset, Rejuvenate
3. Embodiment
4. Alchemy
5. Consciousness
6. Awakening
7. The Body Awakening Method

Combined, this is a bespoke nutritional transitioning cycle. The journey through this sacred body- and life-awakening cycle means trusting nature is your ally, choosing nature as your only operating table. Nature is loving, healing, nourishing, and holds the codes of transformation you are looking for. You must be trusting that you can heal anything, given the understanding of the process of nutritional transitioning, cellular detox, cleansing, herbal regeneration, and healing the trauma stored inside at a cellular level. Accomplishing this can reset the body to its most ultimate state of optimal health.

Step 1—Nature's Natural Rhythms

Nature has rhythms and so does your body, and they are deeply interconnected. When you live in alignment with nature, you attune to the universe. Not only that, you will see your body heal fully, and you come home to you.

To get in harmony with natural rhythms, isolating and combining certain foods is essential. A few things you can do are always eating fruit by itself, not drinking while eating food, keeping food simple, knowing that more fibrous/savoury foods are easier on the body after 3 pm, and that for 12 to 13 hours per day dry, juice, or fruit fasting is a super vibrant full-body reset.

The information shared with the body from nature is that which awakens you back to your five-dimensional soul self, which includes THE HEART as a place and love as where you begin to remember your true self. As the layers of a conditioned life, toxins, emotions, habits, and patterns drop away, and you shed your skin, you experience a rebirth, a renewal. You re-awaken to a higher vibration where you begin to create a more abundant, joyful, aligned, happy, spiritual loving state. This is a peaceful reality, so within, so without, so below, and so above.

Step 2—Cellular Remove, Repair, Reset, Rejuvenate

This is an essential four-step process within the seven steps, which is to totally heal the cells of the body which make up your organs-systems and which are what create your life. Each cell is life, and each cell holds habits, patterns, addictions, residual waste, cravings, and imprints. This is why I talk so much about cellular health. It is so very important, and it really is the most liberating process anyone can ever implement into their life. Cellular health can transform all areas of life and embody real, permanent change. Fad diets are temporary, cellular alkaline living is a real truth.

Eating foods that affect your cellular level allows you to heal your entire digestive system, gut absorption, assimilation, and elimination. After that, your liver, kidneys, endocrine glands, and lymphatic system are helped. This is the missing link for so many. When these systems are healed, repaired, rebuilt, cleaned, and brought back to health, then vitality, strength, and liberation prevail as obstruction is removed and well-being is reinstated into every cell of your BEing.

To eat foods that affect your cellular level start by using high water-content fruits and veggies, greens, herbs, herbal formulas, enemas, fasting, yoga, sex energy, transformation healing, and lymphatic movement. The cells begin to either die off and are eliminated, or they renew and repair. This is a positive transformation, which elevates you to achieve and be more of your full potential.

Step 3—Embodiment

Embodiment is everything. When you embody your truth, when you fully embody your true self, after the layers of toxins have been shed, you will experience a kind of health very few are experiencing, maybe only 1 percent of the people on our planet right now. This is where you will experience permanent results and freedom in your body.

Embodiment comes from *be-ing-in-your-body*. By this, I mean, it's about actually living from your body heart. You have to be present inside yourself with your energy and what lights you up, makes you feel good, and what makes

YOU happy. What do you really want, not getting lost in what everyone else wants around you? What LIGHTS up your SOUL? If you're lit up, you will light up the world, and this is what we need more of.

It takes consistency and responsibility to yourself. When you feel embodied, you feel confident, grounded, centred, clear, calm, peaceful, empowered, like your inner-flame has been switched on, permanently, fully, and completely in alignment. This is where you transcend all limitations, and you align to your divinity, embodying your divine nature in this human body. This is called your zero-point.

Step 4—Alchemy

Alchemy is where you get to transform the old into the new. You get to renew, rebirth, awaken, and rise higher. You can do this by using pure whole foods and mucus-free eating to totally clear the body of all waste. You can apply dry, juice, and fruit fasting, breath work, and transitioning. You can move any old, stuck, stagnant energies which are emotion (e-motion is energy in motion). Alchemy is about more than the transmutation of matter. It is converting old energies into higher energies, and it is why we need light and dark, night and day. It is all wholeness, oneness, a universal elixir to live your best, most awakened life. It's all connected, and nutrition is a sacred, powerful tool of freedom when used correctly.

Step 5—Consciousness

The food you eat is either conscious or unconscious, and it can be very simple. We don't need to kill an animal to survive when we have been provided an abundance of non-animal foods that the human body thrives on. It is no longer about survival. It is about thriving in this body on our sacred planet. You get to choose this every time you eat. I also have deep compassion here. It's not simply about giving up everything. Many human bodies have become so acidic, they crave those acidic animal foods and lots of cooked food, but it isn't necessary. Avoiding acidic animal foods helps you clear the residue, and it is part of your transition.

STEP 6—Awakening

This step is actually the first step in the process that you get to see, feel, and know that you don't need those foods, the animals, who also have feelings and emotions. They feel love, sadness, and fear, just like you. You get to raise your vibration and create a body you feel at total peace in, as you are no longer processing lots of animal emotions and waste not meant for the human body.

I have reached a point where my body has cleared of a lot of waste. Generally, I fast for part of every day. Other times, I only eat fruit and drink fruit juice and herbs, and sometimes I'll spend a whole day doing this. The longest I did was 35 days of just fruit and herb fasting with other support. As already mentioned in this chapter, to support the healing process, I could eat other delicious foods, but my body just loves this deep cleansing so much that life becomes effortless here.

Fruit is one of your most powerful foods for health, when used in alignment with the body and correctly interwoven into your healing process.

Step 7—The Body Awakening Method

YOU awaken to a utopia that starts inside your body. You are the heaven on earth. You have arrived home to your true self, centred, embodied, calm, peaceful, knowing, and deeply awakened as your highest and best version of you. Through the process of elimination, your body makes space to integrate a new energy and structure.

Your body is at least 60 percent water, so with this, you can recalibrate this water daily to a new structure. It's flexible. You get to change and adapt daily. Change is healthy, safe, and feels good. Change is something many people fear, and I did for a long time until I saw change was on my side. Change is supporting you to grow, evolve, and *be more YOU*.

Step seven is the core, the centre of the earth, the heart, unconditional love, and this is exactly where the process takes you—home to your HEART. You arrive home to divinity. You work your way around *The Body Awakening* way, starting at 80/20 alkaline/acid where you may have a vegan pizza or bread or pasta or vegan cheese; to some cooked and lots raw; to all raw veggies and fruits; to just fruit; to mono-fruit eating. It is a process that can be totally be-spoke to you, so you can achieve your highest health and life excellence, living at your full health potential. From juice fasting to dry fasting—dry fasting is the highest of all, where old cells get broken down and moved out of the body, and why you can transform, so I encourage you to fast on dry fasting protocols.

You are literally dissolving the past, the old, and rapidly moving forward to your highest life of bliss, joy, health, wealth, and freedom. It must be done properly, and I always suggest doing it with an expert by your side. I hope this sets a powerful foundation for you to transform and rise and live your BEST, most fulfilled, awakened, and empowered life in a body you love, where you remember and embody your true self, and live your most abundant, happy, and healthy life.

About the Author

Arianna Auñón is an award-winning women's health, thyroid, and cellular detox coach and specialist. She is a healer, intuitive, a retreat facilitator, and a natural health advocate. She is a truth seeker and catalyst to facilitate the awakening of the true health sovereignty of humanity.

With nearly 20 years of life experience, studies, and research on healing, as well as her own journey of all-naturally healing hypothyroid, autoimmune anxiety, stress, emotional eating disorders, addiction, and codependency, Arianna came home to her true self, a soul remembrance. Arianna emanates vibrant health. She is the founder and creatrix of The Body Awakening Method and Barefoot Luxury Alkaline Living, a healing method and way of living that gets to the root cause, sets a powerful foundation for true health, and allows you to live your healthy, empowered truth, embodied and free.

Arianna specialises in hormonal health, thyroid health, gut health, detoxification, weight loss, stress, anxiety, self-esteem, energy, alignment, quieting the busy mind, embodiment, emotional eating, The Feminine Body, true self awakening, coming home to divinity, inner peace, love, bliss, and an opening of the heart. She supports women around the globe to next-level health, body awakening, and true soul remembrance of the true-divine-self, with nature as our ally. Arianna says, "It is here we embody our true divine nature."

Arianna is currently co-authoring a book on health and spirituality, and finalising her own book, *The Body Awakening*. She offers bespoke one-on-one specialist support and The Body Awakening Barefoot Luxury Alkaline Living retreat experiences.

Email: info@ariannaaunon.com
Website: www.ariannaaunon.com

CHAPTER 4
STRESS: THE DRIVER BEHIND CHRONIC DISEASE

By Marian Bourne
Founder, The Bourne Practice for Stress
Management and Health Mentoring
London, England, United Kingdom

The greatest weapon against stress is our ability
to choose one thought over another.
—William James

The word "stress" has become so ubiquitous in our language, that for many people it no longer has much meaning. We say we're stressed when we feel upset, angry, frustrated, overwhelmed, or feel any negative emotion we don't like.

Originally, stress was defined by the "father of stress", Hans Selye, as "the response of the body to any demand, whether it is caused by, or results in, pleasant or unpleasant conditions". That definition is just over 40 years old, but it is no longer considered to be entirely accurate.

Today, we recognise that there are two aspects of stress—stimulus based and response based—and neither can be accurately defined since a stimulus to one person, may be a mild irritation to someone else. Similarly, each person's response to stress differs widely, depending on many different factors in their life.

A stress stimulus can be physical, emotional, psychological, or environmental, for example, the toxic chemicals found in weed-killers and pesticides;

or internal infections that can be hard to diagnose such as yeast, viruses, parasites, bacteria. It can include dental work, for example, amalgam fillings, root canals, extractions. Other stressors include eating a junk diet; having surgery or spending time in hospital; getting injured; being in a car crash; divorce; moving house; or death of people close to you. Most people are not aware that each of these contribute to the body's "burden" of stress.

Emotional stress is probably the type of stress that most people easily recognise. Paradoxically, though, it is often underestimated. When people live with a lot of stressful situations, they learn to adapt, they learn to cope, and they learn to get on with life. After all, stress is good for you, isn't it? Yes, but only up to a point.

People are "programmed" to adapt and cope. Human beings have been "wired" to look out for danger for millennia. Without this ability to look out for danger or adapt to different situations, we would not have survived as long as we have. Given that our survival is dependent on how alert we are to danger, it's not surprising that our neural "wiring" and our adaptive responses to 21st century stress are just as finely tuned (and probably more so) as they were for our ancestors.

Our stress responses are meant to "turn on" for the duration of the stressful event and then "turn off". When our ancestors escaped the proverbial sabre-toothed tiger, their nervous system then had time to reset back to normal once the danger was over.

Unlike our ancestors, many of us live with a 24-hour assault on our nervous system. This is something we weren't designed for. In today's world, we either don't have time to re-set and recover, or worse still, it is no longer recognised as necessary. Indeed, in some business cultures there is a "badge of honour" if you live with and appear to thrive on high levels of stress. The short-term stress when you have time to recover is not a problem. However, when the acute short term becomes the chronic long term—and there is no magic number or marker that will tell you when you have moved from one phase to the next—is frequently when health problems start. In the words of Hans Selye: "It's not stress that kills us, it's our reaction to it".

How we react or respond to stressful situations will be different for each of us. You may find sitting in long traffic queues very stressful—you'll be late, it's a waste of time, you get angry that there are so many cars on the road, you may even feel yourself building up to some form of road rage. Alternatively, your reaction could be one of complete acceptance; You relish this opportunity to listen to some music, think and plan your day ahead. You know that the situation can't be changed, it is what it is and so you see it as an opportunity rather than a challenge.

How you are wired to handle stress will determine whether or not stress affects you negatively. So, the question is, what determines how your nervous system, i.e., your wiring, responds to stress? And is there anything you can do about it? One way of answering this is to say that a lot depends on 1) what happened to you as a child, 2) how you managed or didn't manage to handle it, 3) the number and frequency of stressful situations you have experienced as an adult, and 4) how well you handled them.

What happened to you as a child can range from a "normal" uneventful childhood that had all the usual ups and downs, which you may or may not have coped with well, to traumatic events now known as adverse childhood experiences (ACEs). They include all types of abuse, neglect, incarceration, and domestic violence, as well as parental mental illness.

Whatever happened to you, your nervous system responded. The three most common responses that most of us recognise are fight, flight or freeze. With the first two, you feel activated to take action, literally to fight or run. Your heart rate and breathing rate go up, you have increased blood flow to your arms and legs. With freeze, you may well feel frozen to the spot in difficult or stressful situations, but freeze is also a state that can develop long after a traumatic situation, where you feel a low level of depression and you don't understand why you feel so little motivation to do much of anything.

What's very confusing about your stress response is that you can feel wired up to the national grid and at the same time feel as if you're shutting down. It's as if you have an internal tug-of-war going on inside and you've lost the OFF switch to both. The good news is that you can rewire how your nervous system responds to stress.

Perhaps you've seen diagrams of the nervous system "wiring" in an anatomy book and you've noticed that it runs from the top of the body to your toes and from your skin and organs to your brain. It covers your entire body, like a complex road map that connects everything together. These connections mean that what you do to the body will have an impact on your thinking and behaviour, and what you think and believe will affect your physical body.

In case this concept seems alien to what you know, think about a time you were in love or you passed exams or got your dream job/partner/house. How did you move? How did you sound? What expression did your face show to the world? If good news and excitement can make you smile and change how you move and talk, it's useful to know that at the same time, you're also producing "happy hormones" such as oxytocin, serotonin, and dopamine. Happy hormones influence digestion, sleep and brain function, and even circadian rhythms.

By contrast, when you react negatively to situations, your nervous system is activated to produce a fight, flight or freeze response, and simultaneously, your adrenal glands are stimulated to release adrenalin and cortisol.

Your adrenal glands sit on top of your kidneys, just under the last (twelfth) rib. Even though they are no bigger than a walnut, their impact on your body is significant. Not only do they influence how you think and feel, they influence many physiological processes in your body, such as how you break down carbohydrates and fats; whether you have stored fat around your waist; whether you are prone to allergies; whether you have good control of your blood sugar. After menopause, your adrenals are the major source of sex hormones for both men and women. They're small but mighty powerful!

How many times have you heard of people being prescribed steroids, for example, NSAIDs, by their doctor? They're used to reduce pain and inflammation and to reduce the body's immune response in certain situations. They're often prescribed for skin conditions, such as eczema and dermatitis; for gut conditions, such as Irritable Bowel Syndrome, Ulcerative colitis and Crohn's disease; and for allergies, asthma, injuries, and soft tissue damage, such as tennis elbow or bursitis. A pharmaceutical drug is prescribed because it imitates the actions of your own cortisol and by prescribing it your doctor intends that it will similarly have the same effect. Sometimes this works and sometimes it doesn't. It's useful to know that NSAIDs have side effects.

If you're living with a lot of stress, the likelihood is that you are living with a lot of cortisol. What most people don't realise are the number of different factors that can affect your adrenals and the amount of cortisol you produce. Below are some of these factors, some will be familiar but others might surprise you:

- Emotional stress
- Financial pressure
- Death of someone close
- Fear
- Marital stress

- Exercise—too much or too little
- Allergies
- Smoking
- Divorce
- Lack of sleep
- Bad/poor diet
- Using food and drink as stimulants
- Staying up late despite being tired
- Constantly driving yourself to do better/be better
- Trying to be perfect
- Lack of rest and relaxation
- Very stressful work conditions
- Sugar/refined carbohydrates
- Prescription and non-prescription drugs
- Caffeine—coffee, energy drinks, etc.
- Negative attitudes and beliefs
- Toxicity—amalgam fillings, car exhaust, outgassing from new carpets, curtains and, newly treated wood, yeast infections, parasites, bacterial infections, root canals, pesticides, and fumes from petrol and diesel
- Injuries and accidents

It doesn't matter what type of stress you're subjected to; your body is wired to respond with cortisol. Not only are each of the factors listed above a source of stress, if they are repeated or you are subjected to several at the same time, your level of stress will be greatly increased. Over time, however, your adrenal glands can become depleted and rather than having an excess of cortisol, you have too little. This might mean you have adrenal fatigue, or if your body no longer produces cortisol, you will be diagnosed with Addison's disease.

You might be thinking that we would be better off without cortisol, but we need it for many physiological actions. At the most basic level we need cortisol to stimulate our muscles to run from danger, so you could say, we are no different from a zebra or gazelle that needs to escape from a hungry lion. The only thing that is different today is that we have cortisol responses to so many different things that we find stressful (as listed above), and we don't have time to reset afterwards.

Too much or too little cortisol both cause health problems, which is why it's so important to understand that stress is the number one enemy of health, relationships, and even libido. Luckily, there are usually a number of warning symptoms that help us to recognise when we're having trouble coping with stress. Symptoms are what we sense and feel, and they usually precede the signs, which are visible or are revealed in a laboratory test.

Emotional symptoms include anxiety, irritability, sadness, defensiveness, anger, mood swings, hypersensitivity, apathy, depression, and slowed thinking or racing thoughts.

Physical symptoms include headaches, grinding teeth, clenched jaws, chest pain, shortness of breath, pounding heart, irritability, muscle aches and pains, indigestion, constipation or diarrhoea, increased perspiration, fatigue, insomnia, ulcers, frequent colds, and weight gain.

Social and career changes include increased use of alcohol, smoking, recreational drugs, loss of libido, marital and relationship problems, withdrawal from social situations, rigid thinking, restlessness, and poor job performance.

All of the above symptoms can be recognised if we know what to look for. What can't be seen are the internal changes taking place in the body—increased blood pressure, increased metabolism (e.g., faster heartbeat, faster respiration), changes in intestinal movement (digestion), changes in immune and allergic response systems, increased cholesterol and fatty acids in the blood for energy production, localised inflammation (redness, swelling, heat, and pain), faster blood clotting, increased production of blood sugar for energy, increased stomach acids, increased blood glucose levels, decrease in protein synthesis, and hormone changes affecting thyroid hormones and sex hormones such as oestrogen and testosterone leading to low libido. Unfortunately, it's not always obvious that stress could be at the root of someone's problem.

Mary, 49, couldn't understand why she felt exhausted and could barely get out of bed in the morning. She had a well-paid job and enjoyed it; she was on track to becoming a senior manager in her department. She had no financial worries and a comfortable home and good marriage. On the surface, her life looked very easy and she couldn't see any reason for her exhaustion.

It turned out her mother was ill with cancer, her husband was about to be made redundant, and her eldest daughter had a diagnosis of anorexia. To cope with this, Mary was going to the gym six days a week, snacking on chocolate during the day "for energy", and drinking six to eight cups of coffee a day.

When I asked Mary about any stresses in her life, she told me she had none. Her response was very typical. We get used to what is going on and we adapt, until our body has no more ability to adapt. It's hard for many people to believe that stress might be the root cause of their health problems. They know people who burn the candle at both ends and have buckets of energy; others who seem to thrive on meeting tight deadlines and working round the clock; they know people who are too busy to take holidays and if they do, they're to be seen sitting by the pool answering emails and talking to the office. All these people seem to be "fit and healthy".

For anyone who can't recognise that stress and its accompanying hormone, cortisol, might be involved, I recommend finding and taking an Adrenal Stress Profile Laboratory test, which measures salivary cortisol during the day. You can find out where to take such a test online.

With recognition and awareness of the damage stress can cause, the question now needs to be asked—*how can you stay healthy despite living with a lot of stress?* And similarly—*how can you recover?*

The two approaches will vary, but there are some themes common to both. Below is a five-step process I use to help people who recognise they are not handling stress as well as they would like and who do not want to hit burn out and possibly 'crash'. This process can be remembered by the acronym AWARE.

Awareness
What works
Analyse
Reset
Embody

Awareness—Reality Check-In

Part 1. Awareness is all about doing a reality check-in. I recommend doing a 360-degree examination of the whole of your life. Using a "wheel of life" is a good way to have a visual representation of what your life looks like. You can score your happiness from 1 (very unhappy) to 10 (totally happy). To complete the wheel of life, score each of the following on a scale of 1 – 10. Satisfaction and fulfillment of your career, financial situation, friendships, relationships, health, fitness, fun/relaxation, and family. The visual result from doing a wheel of life can be an eye-opener as to where you might want to make some changes. Even if your happiness level is high, your fulfilment in career is high, financial situation is high, but friendships or relationships are low, there is work to be done!

Part 2. Make a list of everything that has happened over the last 10 years. For example: deaths of people close to you; financial difficulties; changes in working conditions; problems with a difficult boss or colleague; changes in sleeping habits; changes in eating habits; changes in exercise habits; how much fun or relaxation you have per week; trouble with in-laws or family; difficult neighbours; arguments with family, friends, relatives; moving house; difficult health diagnoses; injuries and accidents; marriage; divorce; retirement; and redundancy.

All of these events contribute to your stress levels. Obviously you can't undo or change events in the past, but acknowledging the events you've had to cope with can help you understand the background to your current situation.

What Works—Shine and Show Spotlight

Everyone has coping strategies. It can be difficult to recognise them because they're so much a part of who you are. For example: ignoring your own needs and working harder; eating more than usual or comfort eating; smoking or drinking too much coffee or caffeinated drinks; withdrawing emotionally; ignoring the problem; getting angry for no good reason; sleeping more than necessary; taking time off from work; retail therapy, shopping. When you recognise what your default coping strategies are, you are in a position to change them.

Analyse—Deep Dive Directive

This step isn't easy to do on your own. Essentially, it's a long hard look at the beliefs and patterns of behaviour that have been running your life since you were about seven years old. Sometimes there are beliefs that you may need help to identify. Very often our beliefs are our blind-spots, we don't see them.

Reset—Reset Roadmap

Reset is all about learning to rewire your nervous system to respond differently to stressful situations. This step of learning starts at the outset of following the programme so that you have skills to use immediately, which, over time, become embodied as part of your coping strategies.

Empower—Building Your Blueprint

The skills you learn to handle stress show you how to listen to the messages from your body and teach you what action you need to take. They become a blueprint for feeling deeply connected and centred to your own inner wisdom.

If there is one thing to take away from reading this chapter, it is this: in a world where we are more connected than ever before through the technology available to us, we must make sure not to lose connection to our body's whispers of distress and the voice inside us that speaks through intuition. Our health and well-being are not in the same category of servicing a car or maintaining the antivirus programmes on our computers.

Your body is your connection to the world, it lives and breathes in relationship to your thoughts and beliefs. Stressful situations that trigger changes in your thinking and changes in your cortisol levels, will nearly always have a knock-on effect, albeit subtle, on your physical body. In his book, *When the Body Says No,* Dr Gabor Mate states that stress is the underlying factor in chronic disease. We owe it to ourselves to take as much responsibility as we can for our well-being, and it starts with being aware.

As Danzae Pace says, "Stress is the trash of modern life—we all generate it, but if you don't dispose of it properly, it will pile up and overtake your life."

About the Author

Marian Bourne runs a private Health Mentoring and Stress Management Coaching Practice in London. She works with highly successful women in leadership to reduce stress levels and restore their well-being. Marian's 20-year background of treating chronic health conditions combined with stress management coaching, gives her unusual and valuable skills in preventing high-performing women in leadership from hitting burnout and taking early retirement. She is certified as a senior coach with the IAPC & M; is accredited in Conversational Intelligence®; and has a rich background of specialist therapeutic modalities in healthcare. Marian says, "I know that women in leadership are exceptionally good at keeping commitments to other people, but they're not so good at keeping a commitment to take care of themselves; as a result they pay the ultimate price with their mental and physical health.

Email: marian@thebournepractice.co.uk
Website: www.marianbourne.com
Website: www.thebournepractice.co.uk
LinkedIn: https://www.linkedin.com/in/marianbourne

CHAPTER 5

IF YOU WANT IT, YOU HAVE TO FIGHT FOR IT!

By Kyle Coletti
Owner of Focusmaster Fitness, Winner of SPIKE TV's Sweat Inc.
Clifton Park, New York

Nothing worth having comes easy.
—Theodore Roosevelt

One reason obesity is on the rise in the United States is because, for most people, it's easy to achieve—move less, eat more, and never really get uncomfortable. If you feel like your body has been trending down the wrong path, I'm here to help reroute your journey and give you the little nudge you need to start tackling your health and fitness goals. I'm going to show you how small shifts in your thinking will help you stay on track, so you can become a healthier, more fit version of yourself.

In this chapter, you'll find my own philosophy on fitness, healthy lifestyle habits, and the mindset needed to achieve fitness goals you may currently think are impossible. My philosophy has been developed through an accumulation of years of study as well as my own personal experiences going all the way back to my childhood in a hardworking middle-class family in Troy, New York.

Over the past ten years I've owned and operated Focusmaster Fitness, where I've personally run thousands of fitness classes, created fitness programming for gyms around the world, and earned the title "America's Next Fitness

Phenomenon" for winning a nationally televised TV show called *Sweat Inc.* I've witnessed a wide range of clients with different body types, varying degrees of athleticism, and at different stages of their fitness journey achieve amazing and lasting transformations. These real-life experiences have provided me with a unique understanding of how to help you uncover the source of your frustration, find solutions, and overcome your obstacles. Now let's dig in and see what's been holding you back.

To get to where you want to go, you need to know where you are. Take a minute and be honest with your current situation. If you're not where you want to be, how far away are you? Are you in the worst physical shape you've ever been, or are you just trending toward a place you don't want to be? Maybe you're fairly happy with where you are today but know that you need to establish some healthier habits. Either way, you need to recognize your current situation and then start working backwards to see how you got to where you are today.

I'm going to assume that there isn't just one factor that has led you to where you are now. It's more likely that there is an accumulation of small lifestyle changes that slowly turned into habits and now, after a few years, have become the dominant patterns in your life: having kids, a stressful job, a long commute, an injury that has lingered, money issues, divorce—the list can go on and on. On the surface, all these legitimately describe why you have been putting your own personal health on the backburner, but I'm here to tell you that they are all just excuses. The guy or girl that you see on the cover of the fitness magazine with the abs and chiseled arms likely has kids, has a 50/50 chance of getting divorced, probably has money issues, and most definitely has lingering injuries. So how are they able to be so fit when they face the same obstacles? How do they have the time, motivation, or the drive? The difference is their mindset.

It's pretty simple. The fit individual prioritizes their health. There are endless reasons why, mostly dealing with motivation, which we'll get into in a little bit, but in the simplest form, they've had a shift in their mindset, and they see the world and their challenges or options through a different lens. It consciously and eventually subconsciously becomes part of every aspect of their life. When you look closely, there are never any true "overnight" successes in business. The same goes for most fit people and their own personal fitness journeys. Their bodies, their health, and their fitness levels are the accumulation of thousands of small decisions repeated over time that have led to where they are today.

You have to train your mind to find the answer that will lead you to the healthier outcome. "You don't understand, Kyle, I have a super stressful job," you might argue. My answer is "Great, do you know what helps relieve stress? A good workout."

"My back has been killing me for years, I'm afraid I will just get more hurt," you might say.

So, is living with back pain and getting more sedentary the solution? No.

"Kyle, I'm just so busy. I don't have any time in my day."

Pull up your smartphone and show me how you spent your day. You're honestly telling yourself that you can't find 20 to 30 minutes in your day? Before you ever start to see your body change, you need to begin to make the necessary mental changes to find solutions tailored with your health and fitness in mind.

How do you train your mind? Well, just like any other skill: you have to practice. Start out with the simplest things like choosing to take the stairs instead of the elevator, cutting out the sugar in your coffee, asking your spouse if they want to go for a walk after dinner. At first, you have to do the things you don't want to do. Remember, doing ALL the things you like doing got you to where you are today and that doesn't seem to be working for many people. A coffee with no sugar may not seem appealing today, but do it for a couple of weeks and you'll start to feel like it's not that big of an ask.

Change rarely happens in a "cold turkey," "all or nothing" mentality. It's typically a series of gradual changes that lead to positive results. One good habit leads to another, which leads to another. Compounded over a series of weeks, months, and years, you become a completely different person. You have this ability in you, and I want this chapter to be the spark that ignites your fire.

I have witnessed so many incredible body and life transformations within our amazing Focusmaster Fitness members who have come through our studio over the years. One of those success stories is Angel. Angel started Focusmaster several years ago after she had hit somewhat of a rock bottom, as many of us have, juggling the challenges of life, raising four kids, and trying to just keep her head above water. Her breaking point was one night when she was lying in bed, eating a Snickers bar, and all she could feel was her double chin. She was tired, out of shape, and overweight, and she knew that something had to change. She wanted to be a better role model for her kids, and the only way that could happen would be to start putting some of her priority back into herself. It started with carving out 30 minutes a day only a couple times a week.

As Angel began to feel a little more comfortable, instead of hitting two and three classes per week, she started hitting four and five classes. Just like Angel, once you make the commitment to something, in particular, working out, there is change in perspective you get, a clarity, and you realize that actually feeling better can be more rewarding than looking better. For some, feeling better actually becomes a healthy addiction replacing depression and other unhealthy habits from inactivity to binge eating.

As Angel began to feel better, she also started to see her body change. She started to look at her diet to see what small changes she could start making to propel her transformation.

During a body transformation like Angel's, at first, you begin to notice little changes, almost like compound interest in a bank account. You're working out, you're getting better at the workouts, you start to develop some toned lean muscle that you haven't seen in years, your conditioning gets better, your calorie burn begins to increase, and then you actually begin to find compounded enjoyment in the workouts and the benefits that they provide.

Angel went on to become a Focusmaster diehard, which led her to accepting the challenge of becoming a Focusmaster Coach when the opportunity presented itself. And then, three years after her first day walking into Focusmaster, Angel completed her first marathon. Through this journey she lost a total of 65 pounds. If you would have told her on day one what her next few years would look like, she would have called you crazy! She was lightyears away from the mother who was lying in bed, eating Snickers, and her journey all started with one decision.

Now that you are armed with the knowledge of what a small shift in your mindset can do, you need to understand the power of motivation and how essential it is to helping you stay committed to pursuing your goals. Think of motivation as the gas that feeds your engine. In order to reach your goals, you're going to need to look for it everywhere you can. Some call this their "why"— their driving force that gives them the reason to make the sacrifices, to take on the daily challenges, to keep striving toward their goal. For Angel, it was to be a better role model for her kids. For others, it might be to fit into a pair of old jeans, to look and feel their best for a wedding, or becoming healthier, so they don't have to be on certain medications. I recommend taking a couple minutes and really thinking deeply about what your motivation is. What makes you want to be better, be healthier, to reach your goal? I'm telling you right now, most days you will not want to work out, and you will not want to give up the everyday treats you have become dependent on, so you'll need to keep this top of mind every day.

For me, I try to find motivation everywhere I can. I try to store it in my mind, so when the days come that I just don't feel like doing it, I think back and pull motivation from my memory bank. This immediately shifts my mindset. Whether it's a scene from *Rocky* or an Under Armour commercial, I bottle up that motivation and save it for when I need it.

For the past few years, I've been doing the CrossFit Murph workout with my brother-in-law. The Murph workout involves a one-mile run, 100 pullups, 200 pushups, 300 squats, and then another one-mile run. This past year, I wanted to have completed it, but I didn't really feel like actually doing it. On the morning of our scheduled Murph workout, I was searching for motivation from anywhere I could find it. I ended up watching an Ironman motivational YouTube video before the workout, and I listened to it during the one-mile runs. I know I needed extra motivation on this day that I didn't feel like working out. The messaging in the video was the exact trigger I needed to not only start the workout but to excel at it. I ended up trimming three minutes and 30 seconds from my overall time to complete the Murph workout from the year before. Was the motivation that I was able to muster up the only reason I did so well? Probably not, but I know it helped me push my body the entire time.

Fear can also be a powerful motivator. Maybe it's the fear of ending up like some of your unhealthy relatives. Having to take blood pressure medications or insulin due to years of unhealthy habits. It could be a fear of having to stop an activity you truly enjoy doing, perhaps a sport you would like to continue to play for many years to come. The fear of regret is what often helps me stay motivated at certain times. It allows me to be bolder in my dreams and to take actions to try and reach them. I like to carry this mindset with me: "The fear of not taking the chance is greater than the fear to start." There may come a time where your "why" has faded. It may have passed, like in the situation of a wedding, or it could just be that you've stopped seeing the progress at the pace in which you had hoped. You may begin to feel like you're wandering, and you start asking yourself questions like, "Why am I getting up an hour early each day?" and "Why am I not having ice cream at my son's birthday?" This is all normal. Your reasons will change, your desires will change, and when you feel like you hit this wall it's a good time to take a step back to see what you really want at this point in your journey. There are ebbs and flows, and sometimes you need to hit the reset button. Then your search begins again with a new motivation that will keep you laser-focused.

Results come in many forms, and creating specific goals that can be measured is the best way to set yourself up for success. You want to know exactly what you are working toward, so it's critical that you are very clear on what success is for you. Simply saying, "I want to look better," is a hard goal to measure because it's a feeling and very dependent on your mood for that given day. You want to create goals that are measurable and attainable for a given time period. For example, "I want to lose 20 pounds over the next six months." Considering that you have the weight to lose, this is a very measurable and attainable goal. You'll want to lose about three to four pounds each month so it's very easy to track, and you give yourself a defined timeline that is realistic. Take a minute to write down a few goals you would like to reach in the next six, 12, or 18 months. Do this right now.

During your journey toward this goal, I'm sure you will begin to experience a wide range of benefits, ones that you might have not been so focused on at the start, but nonetheless, benefits that should be recognized. Your goal may have been focused around weight loss, but several weeks in, you start to notice that you are beginning to have more energy, you're feeling a little less stiff, and you're starting to actually feel stronger. Taking a minute when you experience these aha moments is super important. They are mini-victories and validations that you are on the right path. Use them as fuel to continue.

When it comes to goal setting, the simplest thing needed to achieve any goal is discipline and consistency. It is your job to execute the plan, day in and day out. You need to find comfort in the routine and start functioning like clockwork. Look at every decision during your day and ask yourself, "Is this bringing me closer to or further from my goal?" Make more right decisions each day, and it's only a matter of time before the tide turns in your favor.

Working towards a goal rarely comes without a fair share of frustration and obstacles that you'll need to overcome. Obstacles can happen at any time, and it's usually when you feel like you're really starting to hit your stride. It could be a twisted ankle, a pulled muscle, or even the flu. Don't beat yourself up and don't dwell in the negativity. This is just one of many tests that you'll be facing during your journey. Accept the situation, explore opportunities for ways you can modify, and adapt until it's behind you. Use the setback as a way to focus on things you can control. This is where most would quit and maybe where you may have given up in the past, but now with your new perspective, you can use it as an opportunity to recognize your newly developed inner strength and prove to yourself that you have a lot more fight in you than once thought.

Take a few minutes to review your goal, solidify your "why," bottle up as much motivation as you can, and then just start. You don't need some huge elaborate plan set in place before you start. Stop telling yourself, "I'll start on Monday." Just start today. Throw your sneakers on, start moving, start sweating, and start doing. Action and creating the habit of doing are more important than the end result right now. You'll find that some of your best workouts happened on days when you didn't really have a plan until you started.

In my experience, most people love a little challenge and typically rise to the occasion. That said, I challenge you to invest in your own successful body right now. You have the power within you to reach any goal you put your mind to. Use this chapter as a springboard and come back to it when you're feeling like you need a reset. Remember, the road will be challenging, but anything worth having is worth fighting for.

About the Author

Kyle Coletti is one of the owners of Focusmaster Fitness based in Troy, New York. His company created and sells a unique piece of striking equipment used for boxing, kickboxing, martial arts, and fitness training. Kyle is also the creator of the Focusmaster workout, a 30-minute boxing-inspired workout program that was developed in their fitness studio and is used by people around the world. Kyle was the winner of the TV show, *Sweat Inc.* on Spike TV, earning his equipment and program the title of "America's Next Fitness Phenomenon."

Kyle has launched his programs in a number of national fitness chains like Gold's Gym, Powerhouse Gym, and Retro Fitness. He is also the executive director of programming for Tapout Fitness, where he assisted in the creation of their boutique fitness concept, and he develops all their branded fitness classes.

Kyle loves challenges, and he has a challenge for you right now. Go to workoutsbykyle.uscreen.io and use coupon code WORKOUTNOW for a free 30 days. You can pick from hundreds of workout videos ranging from various lengths and difficulty. This site even provides full 30-day workout programs, so all you have to do is hit play and attack each day!

While Kyle's fitness instruction is both face-to-face and online, he lives in Clifton Park, New York, and is married to his wife of 10 years, Jamie. They have two young boys, Donato and Luca.

Email: kyle@focusmaster.com
Website(s): https://workoutsbykyle.uscreen.io/
www.focusmaster.com
www.focusmasterfitness.com

CHAPTER 6
YOUR CHAMPION WITHIN

By Toni Delos Santos
Sport Psychology Coach, Professional Racquetball Competitor
Santa Ana, California

*Success is peace of mind that is the direct result of self-satisfaction in knowing
you did your best to become the best that you are capable of becoming.*
—John Wooden

What do Michael Jordan, Serena Williams, and Tom Brady all have in common? They are all exceptionally talented athletes who have achieved greatness in both their respective sport and life. When we watch them perform, we see the results of the hours and hours of work that they put in both physically and mentally to be able to achieve their highest levels of success. They have all faced adversity and used the same resilience that they developed throughout their lives by implementing strong mindsets and belief systems that we can all learn from to become the best version of ourselves.

Having the right mindset is one of the most important pieces of the puzzle that individuals need to be successful. After reading this chapter, I am confident you will gain valuable insight into how your brain works. Admittedly, you will understand different mindsets, and you will develop the tools to succeed, thus benefiting all aspects of your life.

Mindset is often defined as an attitude, disposition, or mood. Mindset is established based on the beliefs you have formed from experiences in your life or what you have been told in your formative years. These beliefs set the stage for your ability and confidence to reach your full potential.

Stanford professor and bestselling author Carol Dweck has done extensive research on mindset, and she has established that there are two types of mindsets that exist within people: fixed mindset or growth mindset. According to Dweck, "In a fixed mindset, people believe their basic qualities, such as intelligence or talent, are simply fixed traits." She continues, "Alternatively, in a growth mindset, people believe that their most basic abilities can be developed through dedication and hard work—brains and talent are the starting point."

People with a fixed mindset hold on to beliefs about themselves and their value that they are either naturally good or bad at certain skills and will never be able to attain a higher level. When we have a fixed mindset, we have limiting beliefs that were formed subconsciously as a defensive mechanism to help us to avoid feeling rejection and disappointment. These limiting beliefs get in the way of our growth and development. Some examples of a fixed mindset would sound like this:

- *I can't lose weight because my parents are overweight.*
- *My Little League coach told me that I should play year-round or I will fall behind.*
- *I can't do yoga because a coach once told me that I am not flexible.*

The growth mindset, however, is based on the thought that the ability to learn from each situation and move forward to succeed can always improve. With a growth mindset, each setback is a stepping stone that can get you closer to your goal by making adjustments. Some things will come more naturally than others, and with hard work and dedication your ability to improve and reach your goals is within your grasp.

Let's take the limiting beliefs and move them into the growth mindset way of thinking:

- *I can lose weight by eating healthy and exercising.*
- *If I play another sport in the off-season, I will use different muscles. This will reduce my risk of injury, and I will be excited to get back to baseball.*
- *Yoga is great for relaxing after a stressful day, and I can improve my flexibility.*

Yogi Berra once said, "Baseball is 90 percent mental, and the other half is physical." When the game comes down to the wire, I think we can all agree that physical ability is relatively equal for the top athletes in their sport. Why is it that some athletes are clutch while others choke? What is the difference between hitting the buzzer-beater or missing the game-winning free throw? A major difference lies in the player's ability to block out mind chatter, outside distractions, and be completely focused in the moment.

One of the skills that we may be very proficient at is negative self-talk and beating ourselves up when we make a mistake. I mean, how on earth are we going to learn our lesson if we don't punish ourselves? After all, positive self-talk and giving ourselves a break will make us soft, right? As much as that seems logical to many people, negative self-talk only reinforces limiting beliefs and will not help us reach our goal. We would never talk to our best friends the way we talk to ourselves. Could you imagine if a player missed the first of two free throws in a game, and the coach yelled, "You are the worst free-throw shooter I have ever seen!" I am guessing it wouldn't make the player tougher or help them make the next free throw. However, if the coach called out, "Take a deep breath, you got this!" it would allow that player to be more confident and have a much better chance of draining the next one. We must give ourselves permission to be human and understand that there is no failure. There is only feedback.

Kobe Bryant did not beat himself up after making a mistake. He was quoted as saying, "I'm reflective only in the sense that I learn to move forward. I reflect with purpose."

Having the capacity to control our thoughts and emotions is critical for positive affirmation development. If we can control our thoughts, we are inevitably able to control our emotions. Affirmations not only replace negative self-talk, but they create a powerful feeling of solid confidence. Affirmations have the proven ability to rewire our brains by raising the levels of dopamine, a neurotransmitter that is known as the "feel good" chemical, associated with the feeling that you get when you score a goal, close a big sale, or fit into your skinny jeans from two years ago.

- *I am dedicated and excited to practice.*
- *Every day I am getting in better shape.*
- *I am committed to my training.*
- *I am in charge of me!*

Affirmations help purify our thoughts and restructure the dynamic of our brains so that we truly begin to think nothing is impossible ... When we verbally affirm our dreams and ambitions, we are instantly empowered with a deep sense of reassurance that our wishful words will become reality.
—Dr. Carmen Harra

The Brain: Two Hemispheres

The key to any good relationship is the ability to communicate, and our brain is no exception! We have a left hemisphere and a right hemisphere that communicate with each other by sharing information through a network of fibers called the corpus callosum. The left hemisphere is more focused on our past, and its job is to protect us from danger and take care of business. The left is logical. The right hemisphere is our creative side and makes plans for the future and is where our sense of identity lives. The right is relational.

Al Sargent, author of *The Other Mind's Eye: The Gateway to the Hidden Treasures of Your Mind*, and Marilyn Sargent, business consultant and life strategies coach, pioneered the field of study known as Hemispheric Integration™. They discovered that when we visualize or imagine, each side of the brain has its own unique cognitive style of processing. We each have a dominant hemisphere in which we first process information. Being aware of which side you process information, or lead with first, is a helpful tool to understand the best way to be in charge of motivating yourself.

If you are wondering which is your primary hemisphere, meaning which hemisphere you process information in first, do the following exercise:

First, clasp your hands together with your fingers intertwined and notice which thumb is on top. Now, reclasp your hands, interlacing your fingers this time by putting the opposite thumb on top. Notice how awkward it feels. This physical structure of thinking is similar to having a dominant hand to write with in the sense that both attributes are hard-wired in our brain. Since we all have both a right and left hemisphere of our brain, it is important to gather the information from each side to be in alignment. Sometimes we only pay attention to one side of the brain, and we miss the continuum of processing that goes from right to left or left to right. If we don't honor both sides, we end up saying things like, "I have only half a mind to ...!" which can lead to trouble!

Now about the hands. Do you want to see how they relate to which hemisphere is dominant for you?

- If your left thumb is on top, you are a right brain lead, which means that you learn by making a big picture and then filling in the details.
- If your right thumb is on top, you are a left brain lead, which means you like to have the details first and then you get the big picture.

Example of a right brain lead:

- Invitation: "Want to go to a concert on Friday night?"
- Response: "Yes, that sounds really fun!" Overall big picture, no details needed.
- Example of a left brain lead:
- Invitation: "Want to go to a concert Friday night?"
- Response: "Where is the concert? Who is performing? What time is the concert?" There are no details provided, which are needed before this person can feel safe agreeing.

Understanding which hemisphere we lead with is very helpful in the way we set up our goals. Let's look at an example of setting up the same goal from the left brain lead and the right brain lead.

- Right Brain Lead: I like to travel. I want to go on vacation to Hawaii. I can imagine how much fun it will be to lie on the beach drinking a Mai Tai.
- Left Brain Lead: I want to go on vacation to Hawaii. I am going to have to save money for the airfare, ask for time off at work, and start going to the gym. I can imagine how good it will be to lie on the beach drinking a Mai Tai.

Now that you have your goal and vision in place, the next step is to implement your strategies. However, sometimes a little nagging voice in your head starts to question your ability and resilience to reach your goal. This creates doubt, leading to indecision and often procrastination or even giving up. Confused internal voices can be dangerous.

Examples of confused internal voice:

- "Part of me wants to go to the gym, and the other part wants to sleep in."

- "Part of me wants to save money, but part of me thinks it won't happen because I like to go shopping."
- "Part of me wants to go to Hawaii, but the other part thinks my boss won't let me take time off at work, so why even try?"

What is the driving force behind this voice? Why does part of you think one way and the other part another way? Our perspectives are influenced by experiences, traumas, outside influences, and education. We now know that we have two hemispheres in our brain, each with its own cognitive style, and it is most important that we bring both sides into agreement to achieve success. Determine what is possible by building confidence and finding the truth to update limiting beliefs so that we are creating the same vision from both sides of our brain in order to experience optimum success. This is called being "congruent" or "aligned" within yourself, which is a solid and powerful place to begin facing the world.

Al and Marilyn Sargent teach people how to use the tools of Hemispheric Integration to determine first which hemisphere is dominantly seeing the first image. Finding out what is in the other mind's eye will allow you to make sure you are aligned with your vision, or not. Learn to be a good detective to discover how each side of the brain thinks about your goal in order to understand what has to be updated or brought into alignment, so both sides come into agreement on the same compelling image. Any incongruence or argument within yourself can cause feelings of confusion, depression, or being stuck, which can lead to sabotaging your goal.

Here is an example of using Hemispheric Integration to find out how each side of the brain thinks about your goal of going on vacation to Hawaii.

First, take a deep breath and look out into the distance as if your eyes are a projector. Now, when you think about going to Hawaii, what image do you see? The image will represent how this side of your brain is thinking. Think about:

1. Visual—is the image in color or black-and-white? Movie or still photo? Any other important visual component?
2. Auditory—are there any sounds coming from the image? What thoughts or comments are you saying to yourself as you look at the image?

3. Kinesthetic—what are the physical feelings in your body as you look at the image? It could be tense in your shoulders, relaxed in your gut feeling, tight in your throat, all depending on the content of the image.
4. Meta—now check for your overall emotional feeling or evaluation of what this image means to you. For instance, "I feel happy, excited, angry, calm, scared, etc."

Next, get a sense of which eye you are seeing the image out of. Please note that as you are learning this process, at first you may have to make your best guess. Then, set this image off to the side for a moment and take a deep breath. Gently cover this eye with your hand and ask again, "When you think about going on vacation to Hawaii, what image comes up from this other perspective?" Go back through steps from the original question to thinking about the four aspects of visual, auditory, kinesthetic, and meta. Once you see the image from both sides of the brain, you can identify the parts that may be holding you back and gather the information and resources needed to update any limiting beliefs. This will evolve into a new image to be seen from both hemispheres, so you have a clear picture of the goal you want to achieve, and you can create your strategy for success!

Now that you understand more about the two hemispheres, effectively using your images to work for you can make all the difference in how you motivate yourself to reach your goals. Many times, people come from a place of only moving AWAY from what they don't want to happen as opposed to also moving powerfully TOWARDS what is wanted. An example would be telling yourself, "I don't want to be fat." In this case, all you can see is a picture of yourself overweight. If you don't want to be fat, what *do* you want to be? "I want to be lean and fit" is a better way to look at it. In this case, you can get an image of what that looks like and your body will go towards what is most wanted. In sports, you don't hear a good coach yelling, "Don't strike out!" or "Don't drop the ball!" Instead you hear, "Get a base hit" or "Catch the ball!"

Mental skills, as with physical skills, take time to develop and the more you practice the new skills and techniques discussed in this chapter, the more proficient you will become. Being aware of the many factors that we are in control of to create a positive growth mindset will truly put you on the pathway to success in all areas of your life. You can't ask Alexa for a successful body, and you can't order one on Amazon. The good news is that it is up to you. Only *you* can create your very own champion within.

About the Author

Toni Bevelock Delos Santos is the founder of 90% Mental, a sport psychology coaching company created to assist athletes in unlocking their true potential while developing mental toughness. Passionate about sports, Toni was a world-class professional racquetball player spanning two decades. Her skills in sport psychology and experience as an elite athlete have given her a unique perspective on how to help clients perform under pressure while reaching individual goals.

Toni earned her degree in business administration and marketing at the University of Memphis where she held the title of #1 Woman's Singles Racquetball Player for four consecutive years. Toni also won 10 national titles, and as a member of the US team during the same span, she led the team to seven world championships. In 1988, Toni was honored by the US Olympic Committee and named Athlete of the Year. She now lives in southern California where she enjoys spending time with her husband and two boys, Kai and Dylan.

Email: tonimentalgame@gmail.com
Website: www.90percentmental.com

CHAPTER 7

OLYMPIC WEIGHTLIFTING AND MENTAL TOUGHNESS

By Laura Eiman (interview by Erik Seversen)
Gold Medal Olympic Weightlifter, Mental Toughness Coach
Boynton Beach, Florida

When I first spoke with Laura Eiman, I knew I wanted her message to be included in *The Successful Body* book. A tribute to dedication and mental toughness, Laura, who has received endorsements from icons including Oprah, Rachael Ray, and Barbara Walters, informed me that she loved my book project, but her schedule didn't allow her the time to write the chapter. Always able to find a way, we agreed to an interview chapter. Below is the edited version of my (ES) conversation with Laura Eiman (LE) on August 31, 2020.

Erik Seversen

ES: Hello, Laura. I'm really excited you're speaking with me today. I'm excited to learn even more about your extraordinary life and your perspective on health and the human body. I think the readers of *The Successful Body* are going to benefit from your experience as a gold medal Olympic weightlifter and mental toughness keynote speaker and coach. A quick question that I'd like to start off with is, how did you get started weightlifting?

LE: It was totally by chance. This crazy adventure began first with me doing CrossFit at the age of 60 in Boston. I'd never even seen a barbell before, and, honestly, I thought squats were some kind of Southern vegetable! No kidding. I had zero idea what "functional fitness" was and had never heard of the sport Olympic weightlifting. I was kind of fascinated by the CrossFit culture, and well … all those hard bodies, so I started doing the workouts. I was the oldest one at my local CrossFit box by about 30 years. It took me a long time to drink the Kool-Aid, as they say, and become addicted because I was so out of sync with all the super fit young members cranking out deadlifts and wall balls. The squats were impossible for me and lifting a 15-pound training barbell over my head took about a year to do correctly. But I stuck with it.

In CrossFit, we do two Olympic weightlifting moves: the clean-and-jerk and the snatch. I was really bad at those lifts. They are very precise, difficult moves. When I moved to Florida two years later, I joined a CrossFit gym that had an Olympic weightlifting coach on staff.

I really wanted to improve these two moves, not hurt myself, and develop my own hard body. So, on Saturday mornings, I started taking their Olympic weightlifting classes. I remember like it was yesterday. At my first class, I got cold feet. I looked at the barbell and said "You're not very pretty to look at. In fact, you're kinda ugly, and you seem to be loaded with testosterone. Why on earth would I want to get to know you better?" That barbell literally spoke back to me, I'm not kidding! It said that it could take me to a higher level of mental toughness, a much higher level of focus, calm, and confidence. It would teach me how to keep my ego in check, stay humble, and be positive when the lifting gets scary-heavy. I signed up for an eight-week package of classes, and the next thing you know, a girl next to me throws me her old pair of lifting shoes and says, "You'll need these. Those CrossFit sneakers won't get you anywhere on this platform." The rest is history.

ES: Wow, Laura. That's amazing. So, if somebody else were to try to get started in this, what's your advice for them? You kind of stumbled upon it. What if somebody were intentional? They decided, "I want to get involved in some sort of fitness." What would you say for them to get started?

LE: For anyone wanting to start weightlifting, it's important that you do so safely and correctly right from the beginning. Whether it be lifting a barbell, a kettlebell, dumbbells, or just using your body—sit-ups, pushups, etc., get expert coaching at the start. Weightlifting is a powerful way to get healthy and fit, if it's done correctly. Also, it's important to learn right from the start that it's not about how much weight you are lifting. Even if you're lifting a three-pound dumbbell, you can get great results *if* you are using the proper technique.

Also, this is super important: Find a certified weightlifting coach who will teach you how to breathe correctly and how to control your attitude. It is a huge part of lifting successfully. Many coaches don't bother teaching positive mental attitude, and I think it's a huge void in their program.

ES: That's great advice, and on that note, at the pinnacle of your competition phase, we're not talking about the casual lifter now; we're talking about you competing for a gold medal, getting ready for Olympic weightlifting competition. What is your workout regimen like for something that big?

LE: I am not going to sugarcoat it. It was grueling. I was training at a very elite level. Imagine this: I was in Florida training in a converted garage kind of gym. It was grungy, had no air conditioning. It was 95 degrees and disgustingly humid. It had one floor fan. My routine was a three-hour training session. It was physically one of the toughest things I've ever done. A lot of the time, it was not fun.

ES: And how many days?

LE: At my age I could not train five days a week. My recovery day, my day off, was as important as my training day. (Listen up all you aggressive weightlifters in training. Your recovery day is the time when your muscles are actually repairing and getting stronger, not when you are crushing a PR deadlift. You NEED that downtime!) I was training three days a week. I wanted to do four, but I wasn't recovering fast enough, and I didn't have the energy I needed to perform these explosive moves. I couldn't go into a training session gassed, so my coach and I decided I would train three days a week. It was magic. I got stronger and started to win competitions.

My first 30 minutes is stretching, stretching, stretching, and getting my heart rate up on the rower. Then I would do a full hour of "programming," my coach's specific training plan to get me peaking in my performance at a certain meet. We would train five to six months out for a competition. So, no kidding, his program for me six months out was very specific, so that my strength, my energy level, and the amount of weight I was lifting would peak on competition day. While it was boring and very lonely at times, there was also exciting stuff going on in that oven-hot garage!

Training is very strategic and very precise. The OCD Laura loved the precision of it all. Sports are intense when you're competing at an elite level. So, I would do my coach's programming for an hour and then spend about 45 minutes doing strength and conditioning moves: the grind of pushups, pullups on the rig, weighted squats. Lots of grueling muscle-building exercises, and then I'd cool down for 30 minutes. It's a full three hours when I went to the gym.

ES: Wow! That's amazing. And through all of that, you mention the grueling part about it. So, in your opinion, is the physical or the mental more important for success in weightlifting?

LE: Well, there's no question about it. You *have* to be physically fit to successfully weightlift. Getting fit is a very slow process. It's a six-month, 10-month, 12-month build, depending on what your goals are. I didn't really develop super strong muscles for the first two to three months. But once I got on that training trajectory, I began to respect the process and settled in for the long haul. I just do the work. And then, of course, I had to get my diet, my sleep routine right and cut out all alcohol. So, the physical piece has got to be in place.

But then, the most important piece is getting your mindset straight. It's critical for me to be able to walk into that gym every day and say, "Yes, I can, I believe in myself. I'm excited to be here today. I can lift that barbell today, and I'll lift better and cleaner today than I did yesterday." If I didn't do that, I'd have lost before I even walked in the door.

Now I've seen a lot of really strong athletes in my weightlifting days at the gym, and they're muscling through some pretty impressive lifts, but then I see them crash and burn, especially in competitions, because they don't have the mindset piece mastered. They're using brawn; they're only using their muscle, not using their mind to lift intelligently, and they end up psyching themselves out. They let their big ego get involved, or they don't believe they can do it at all. All sorts of toxic thinking is going on in their heads, and what happens? They don't place on the platform.

I'm going to say that in the end, your physical fitness is critical, and you have to be paying attention to dieting correctly and sleeping correctly. But, at the end of the day, the big perspective, the big picture, it is 20 percent physical, 80 percent mental.

ES: Wow, amazing. Is there a tip that you could give somebody to get into that correct mindset? Is there a mental strategy, or is it just that you either fall in love with weightlifting and you dive in, or you don't?

LE: Yes: "Think about what you are thinking about." This tip is part of my overall strategy for winning. Our thoughts dictate our habits, and our habits form our lives. If you want to change your body and become healthy and fit, it's not primarily about doing that new fad diet or extreme fitness program. You must start by what you feed your mind. You have to begin by getting your thoughts right.

If you could see your thoughts about your body and your lifting practices projected on a jumbotron in Times Square, what would they say to you? Would you feel proud, mortified, happy, or sad seeing them? So many people I talk to literally hate their bodies and tell me they are terrible at golf, at skiing, or at whatever … and then they wonder why they are not achieving lifelong fitness and weight loss results. It's because they are feeding their minds with negative self-thoughts and huge doubts about themselves.

You can't win at anything with a losing mindset. The first step to winning a successful body is to become aware of what you are thinking about. Then the next step is to develop a mentally tough, success-based mindset and replace those toxic thoughts with some big, juicy, happy dreams. Only then are you ready to go after it and get that gorgeous, fit, successful body.

ES: That is really good advice. And how about age? I am 51. I've been told by peers recently, mostly by people a few years older than me, that I'm going to start slowing down. How does someone continue a regimen of fitness as a person ages?

LE: I don't believe in walking on eggshells about getting older. People love to coin phrases and say, "I'm not getting older, I'm getting bolder." Well, that's really cool. I mean, that's lovely, but you know, you're getting older, and I'm getting older, and the most important thing is accept that fact, but then stay in a solution-based, positive mindset about it. Dump the negative beliefs, and consider to yourself at 51, your body is different today than it was when you were 45. How is it different and what are your goals going forward and what kind of activities do you love to do that you can go after? What do you want to do physically in the next five years? What do you want to do for the next 35 years? Then adjust your workout and get going. I've had to. I'm 67 now and I've had to adjust my workout radically in the last two years, because my body has changed. So, I've accepted that and then I've said, "OK, here's what I want to do and here's how I'm going about doing it." I may never be able to swing kettlebells anymore because my lower back is giving me a hard time. But you know what, that's fine, and there are about a hundred other excellent things I can do if I can't swing kettlebells. Adjust and go.

ES: Absolutely. I love that. Earlier, you mentioned a few things about diet. What do you think is the most important thing somebody can do to improve their health through the foods they eat?

LE: Food wise, my immediate reaction is to say, "Get off the sugar and the processed foods." But most people know that by now, so why don't we? Well, these foods are powerfully addictive and toxic and cheaper than eating healthy foods. So, my response is: people should first start feeding their minds with healthier thoughts and stop thinking right away about some new fad diet. I know so many people with good intentions that say, "I'm going to eat healthy on New Year's Day. I'm going to start this diet routine," and then they tank three months in. Why did they tank? Because they haven't developed a positive "Oh, yes I can" mindset to get them through the tough times. Then they tank, feel like a failure, and end up gaining all the weight back, plus 10. Then they tell me that diets don't work. I say, "Well, diets do work. It's people that don't work. It's our mindsets that are not working." So, I'd say, you've got to start first feeding your mind with positive thoughts.

And again, that's my whole coaching program, my Mental Toughness four-step program. I teach people how to change their toxic thinking to positive thinking and how to live in a success-based mindset. It's not easy. It is really, really hard to shift your mindset. I put people through a tough long-term workout of mental pushups. It's very hard work to do, but the most rewarding work you'll ever do is to shift your mindset.

ES: I've heard that from other top-level people. They could usually identify when there was a shift to their mindset and everything turned around, and they went from a life of even struggling health problems to absolute happiness, success, and positive health. I think you mirror a few other really successful people on that.

LE: I am a living example. My life wasn't together for decades and 20 years ago, I had to make a decision. I said, I've got to get mentally tough and learn how to develop a positive mindset because I was not winning at much of anything! To make it worse, I was bingeing on sugar. I should be dead today, but I cut out the sugar 20 years ago. I haven't had any desserts, candy bars, not even Mom's apple pie at Thanksgiving since May 20, 2000. I mastered my emotions. And my mental toughness approach is not about going into some kind of emotional straight jacket and saying, "I'm not allowed to ever be angry. I'm not allowed to ever cry or have a bad day." Of course you are, but the trick is you've got to ask yourself how long do you want to stay in that state? You can stay in that state for five days, five weeks, five years. It depends. You don't have to. You can feel the feelings, then dump them and move on. It takes a lot of practice.

ES: I love the idea of helping others, and it's a win-win all around. What concluding advice would you give to the readers of *The Successful Body*?

LE: I would say, dear reader, you cannot imagine in your wildest dreams how much your life will improve if you treat your body with love and respect. If you want a successful body, my advice is if you really want to 20X your potential and start to win in your life, you don't have to lift heavy objects over your head like I do. You don't have to become a radical vegan or do 21-day juice fasts to feel and look excellent and be happy. First, start to focus on what you're thinking about, develop a can-do positive attitude, and then back it up every day with small action steps. Do that one percent action step every day and imagine where you'll be in 60 days. You'll be 60 percent further along in your health and wellness than you were before you started. Never give up. Never give up.

About the Author

Laura Eiman is a gold medal Olympic weightlifter, Navy SEAL trained "Unbeatable Mind" Certified Coach, corporate consultant, brand ambassador, and keynote speaker. She teaches women in the corporate and college sectors how to develop the mindset of a Navy SEAL and create the habits of Olympic athletes, so they can win at work and in their academics. Laura is also the founder and CEO of PicPads, a company that has garnered endorsements from Oprah, Rachael Ray, and Barbara Walters.

Email: info@lauraeiman.com
Website: www.LauraEiman.com

CHAPTER 8
GROWING OLD THE HEALTHY WAY

By Patricia Faust, MGS
Brain Health Coach, Gerontologist, Neuroscience and Wellness
Lawrenceburg, Indiana

Laughter is timeless. Imagination has no age. And dreams are forever.
—Walt Disney

The Aging Body

As we age, our body goes through somewhat of a metamorphosis. We can see these changes occurring throughout the years, but we are still unnerved when we look in the mirror and that young, fresh face is no longer looking back. The changes are gradual, and we don't really pay attention and notice what is happening until we see the changes. We see gray hair or thinning hair. It seems that our arms aren't long enough anymore to be able to read a menu without glasses. We start to experience weight gain in all the wrong places. Wrinkles and saggy skin drive a huge cosmetic market. None of us wants to look old. As much as we don't want to admit it, we can't hear as well as when we were younger. Hearing loss is now an aging issue. More serious changes that affect our body function include loss of flexibility, muscle strength, and decline in muscle mass. Our metabolism slows down and suddenly we feel OLD!

You can see physical aging and understand what is going on. That can spur you to make changes in your life to maintain a younger physical presence. The point I am trying to make is that when we see and understand that our body is aging, we can take some control to do the best we can to maintain a successful body, even as we age.

The Aging Brain

Now, let's consider our aging brain. Up until the recent past, we believed that our brain produced new neurons (brain cells) and neural pathways until we were in our mid- twenties. Then our brain was fixed, and it just continued to decline throughout our lifetime until we died. This changes when Michael Merzenich of the University of California, San Francisco, Carla Shatz of Stanford University, and Eve Marder of Brandeis University were awarded the Nobel Prize for their discovery of neuroplasticity, also known as the ability of the brain to adapt to the environment. Our brain is capable of new cell growth (neurogenesis), and new connections (neuroplasticity). It has taken some time, however, to determine how we can use these findings to keep our brains young and sharp until the day we die.

Here is the conundrum—we cannot see how our brain is aging and those changes can dictate what kind of life we are living. Our aging brain starts its downward slide in our mid-twenties. Cognitive decline begins to happen. Cognitive function encompasses thinking, memory, decision-making, planning, and speed of processing. Speed of processing is simply quick thinking. I went back to graduate school when I was 50. My classmates were mostly around 25. They were at their peak of cognitive function, and I was at my first acceleration point of cognitive decline. The professor would ask a question of the group, and they would all be giving immediate answers while I was sitting there trying to figure out what the question was. I seriously thought I was nuts to be going back to school. I didn't realize at that point how magnificent my brain was back then. After a few weeks, I was keeping up with everyone else. My brain adapted to my environment and my speed of processing had increased significantly.

The Reasons for Decline

There are many reasons why our brain declines as we age. The brain shrinks through aging. We lose neurons and neural connections as we get older. One of the main reasons is that we don't use them. It is the old "use it or lose it" situation. Our brain is very efficient at pruning cells and connections we don't use. It is constantly striving for efficiency. We become victims of noisy processing in this aging process. Our channels for sensory input, primarily hearing and visual input, deteriorate. If we don't get that taken care of through glasses and hearing aids, our brain struggles to determine what we are hearing and seeing. And then there is weakened neuromodulatory function. This simply means that we are not producing enough brain chemistry (neurotransmitters and hormones) to facilitate brain function.

These aging brain changes can really impact our life, but our brain does not know how old we are. Our brain ages by the lifestyle that we lead. In fact, the World Health Organization, National Institute of Health, and the Alzheimer's Association have all determined the individual risks of certain lifestyle diseases pose an aggregate percentage of risk of developing dementia to be 70%. There are actually some lifestyle barriers that prevent us from having a healthy brain.

Barriers to Healthy Brain Aging

Inactivity is a widespread problem in all age groups. Sitting behind a computer, a TV, or a game console for six to eight hours per day puts you at high risk for dementia. Sedentary lifestyles are epidemic and are as dangerous as smoking a pack of cigarettes a day.

Type 2 diabetes has also become epidemic in the United States. It causes serious damage to the brain. Over time, you are at increased risk of damaging the small blood vessels in the brain. This damage affects the brain's white matter. White matter is the part of the brain where nerves talk to each other. When these nerves are damaged, we end up disrupting our thinking abilities and ultimately cause vascular cognitive impairment or vascular dementia.

Obesity is another chronic condition that puts us at a very high risk for dementia. Obesity does not exist on its own. With it comes a higher risk of high blood pressure, cardiovascular problems, diabetes, and other chronic conditions. All these conditions increase the risk of developing dementia.

Cardiovascular disease is also a problem. The heart and the brain are intimately connected. The prefrontal cortex of the brain is located right behind our forehead. This is the executive function center of the brain, and is involved in rational thinking, decision-making, and cognitive activities. It is an energy cannibal. However, the brain doesn't have its own energy source for the prefrontal cortex to function. Instead, 20 percent of the blood, carbohydrates, and oxygen from each and every heartbeat go directly to the brain. This three-pound organ sitting between your ears uses more energy than any other organ in the body. If we suffer from any type of heart problem, including congestive heart failure or coronary artery disease, the heart is not able to send enough blood, carbohydrates, and oxygen to the brain, and the prefrontal cortex does not function at full capacity.

Untreated hearing loss is a newer addition to the barriers to a healthy aging brain. When we have difficulty hearing, we cannot send clear signals to the brain. When this happens, we increase cognitive load. Cognitive load is increased when unnecessary demands are imposed, therefore, making the task of processing information very complex. I previously stated that as we get older, our speed of processing decreases. We have a hard time remembering information that is complex. Untreated hearing loss makes this situation worse. Our brain slows down even more to decipher the fuzzy signal that it receives when we don't hear clearly. This, again, increases the risk for developing dementia.

Isolation is something else that can produce negative effects on the body. It is especially detrimental to brain health because we are hardwired to connect. This means that we are recipients of DNA hardwiring from our prehistoric ancestors. We are meant to be with other people. When we don't see anyone or talk to anyone over a period of time, our cognitive skills decline.

These barriers seem grim when you are talking about extended lifetimes. Remember that your brain does not know how old you are. It ages in accordance with the lifestyle that you lead. And, we have the power to change our lifestyle, which, in turn, changes our brain. There is hope.

The Healthy Brain Lifestyle

Can you even imagine what it must be like to go through these cognitive declines and believe there was nothing you could do about it? Up until the recent past that was the belief. Dr. Michael Merzenich, a neuroscience researcher, didn't believe that we were doomed to brain decline. Dr. Merzenich is credited as being one of the discoverers of neuroplasticity. This is the ability to make new neural connections that can change our brain. Through neuroplasticity, our brain adapts to our environment—good or bad.

We have the power to change our brain, and we have to be conscious of what we are adapting to. Our brain is naturally in the negative or cautionary state because it has been charged with our survival. It is always on alert for conditions that might harm us. When we don't challenge that perspective, our brain will stay in a negative state. Since we now know that we can change our brain, we can work on being positive. It has to be intentional so that we can focus on the positive side of life. Through repetition and consistency of action, we can create new neural pathways. When we continually respond to the environment in a positive way by the thoughts we think or the actions we take, that neuronal pathway's signal increases in strength to the point that we no longer have to 'think' about the thought or action. We have created a new neural pathway that is so strong it has fallen below the level of our conscious brain to the subconscious brain. This is the beauty of neuroplasticity - we can change our brains.

The other physiological event that can keep our brain young is neurogenesis. This is the ability of our brain to grow new brain cells. This was a major discovery because the belief was that we lose cells as we age, but we never create new neurons. There are certain parts of the brain that are hit especially hard with cell loss. The prefrontal cortex, the executive function center of the brain, and the hippocampus, the center of learning and memory, are especially vulnerable to cell loss. Through neurogenesis, these two areas are able to create more brain volume.

When we grow new cells and connections, we are adding to our cognitive reserve. When we are young, our brains are erupting with massive cell and neural connection growth. We have more than enough to keep our brain functioning on a high level. But around our mid-twenties, that massive growth slows down and then starts to decline. Our brain is losing cells and connections through the type of lifestyle that we live. We don't notice those declines because we have this reserve of cells to take up the slack. When we start to hit our forties, the brain reserve is now becoming depleted. And we start to notice the aging changes. A common one is the tip-of-the-tongue phenomenon. We know a person's name or a word we want to use, but we can't get it out. The more we try to remember, the more likely we won't be able to. A few hours later, that name or word will pop up in our thoughts. Our job at this point is to start replenishing our cognitive reserve. And we can do that by living a healthy brain lifestyle. Each part of this lifestyle contributes something different to our brain function. It is necessary to incorporate all six healthy components given below into your daily life.

Physical Exercise

Our brains are hardwired to move. This was another DNA hardwired gift from our ancient ancestors. There are very critical brain benefits we acquire when we get up and moving. Our brain, specifically our prefrontal cortex, is an energy cannibal. Our prefrontal cortex uses a lot of energy quickly when we are actively involved in thinking, decision-making, planning, and other cognitive functions. You have probably experienced the extreme fatigue when you have had to do a lot of mental work. When we move, our heart beats faster and sends 20 percent of carbohydrates, oxygen, and blood from each heartbeat directly to our brain. We think more clearly, are more creative, and we can be more productive when we give our brain the power it needs to function.

Exercise has more than one benefit. When we exercise, we trigger a protein, brain-derived neurotrophic factor (BDNF) that stimulates the growth of new neurons. It then protects these new brain cells as they mature. This is neurogenesis at its finest.

The physical exercise that you choose to do doesn't have to be over-the-top strenuous. Walking 30 minutes a day, at a moderate pace, for four to five days a week will do just fine. If you can't walk, you can do chair exercises, swimming, or any other aerobic activity that gets your heart beating faster.

The brain benefits of exercise include:

- Better brain function
- Better mental health
- Reduced risk of cognitive decline

Mental Stimulation

We must challenge our brains. Our purpose in learning or experiencing something new is to send new signals to our brain. Our brain is electric and when we stimulate neurons with continual new signals, they start to act together. What fires together, wires together. Finally, we create a new connection. We need to use all the new cells that we created with all our physical exercise. Learning a new instrument or a new language, going to new places, and learning about new cultures are a few ways to energize your brain and make new neural connections.

The brain benefits of mental stimulation include:

- Building stronger brains
- Building positive cognitive reactions from rich lifetime experiences
- Building cognitive reserves: the brain's resilience or ability to cope despite damage or degeneration

Nutrition

Our brain is very specific about its nutritional requirements. Our diet impacts our mental health and well-being. The Alzheimer's Association is championing the MIND diet as a means to slow brain aging, protect against Alzheimer's disease and dementia, and help prevent depression and anxiety. Here are the basics of what a brain healthy diet consists of:

- Time to say no to all that red meat.
- Say yes to lots of green, leafy vegetables and dark red fruits—antioxidants.
- Eating cold-water, fatty fish. Salmon, tuna, and mackerel should become your favorite foods. Baked or grilled.
- Omega-3 fatty acids—there is still a question out about the effectiveness of Omega-3 fatty acids supplements for brain function. It is best to get them through food sources.
- Dark chocolate has flavonoids, antioxidants which protect the brain and the heart.

The brain benefits of nutrition include:

- Positive mental health and well-being
- Slowing of brain aging and protections against Alzheimer disease and dementia

Socialization

Our brain has a fundamental need to connect. This is another case of hard-wiring passed on to us from our ancient ancestors. Social connection is a perception that we are cared for, have assistance available from other people, and are part of a supportive social network. Research shows that being connected protects the brain against the risk of developing dementia and improves mental health and well-being.

Interacting with other people may build cognitive reserves. Social interaction involves many cognitive functions: thinking, feeling, sensing, reasoning, and intuition.

The brain benefits of socialization include:

- Protecting the brain against the risk of developing dementia and improving mental health and well-being
- Building cognitive reserves
- Increasing our cognitive abilities

Sleep

Sleep is a newer addition to the healthy brain lifestyle profile. The research that supports sleep has shown us that our brain is very active while we are sleeping. The newer evidence shows that sleep is required for neuroplasticity and helps flush toxins from the brain. Sleep, including napping, promotes memory formation, and it moves memory from short-term to long-term memory.

While we sleep, we have the glymphatic system give our brain a good scrubbing and cleaning. The glymphatic system is composed of glial cells and cerebral spinal fluid. Cell debris can accumulate through wear and tear, and free radical damage. Our environment poses a risk for toxin buildup in our brain. A deep sleep can allow the glymphatic system to clean our brain.

The hippocampus is the center of learning and memory. When an electrical signal comes in for memory formation, it is transported to the hippocampus for consolidation or encoding. This happens while we sleep.

The brain benefits of sleep include:

- Flushing toxins and debris from our brain by the glymphatic system
- Encoding or consolidating our memories by the hippocampus.

Stress

Stress is our response to a real (or imagined) threat or challenge. Our stress response involves our body, mind, emotions, and thought processes. Stress is so powerful that it can completely negate all the healthy lifestyle changes that we incorporated to change our brain. Stress is something that should not be ignored.

Stress starts and stops in our brain. Remember that our brain is always on alert to stressful or threatening situations. This is critical to our survival. Once more, the stress response was a hardwired gift passed on to us from our ancient ancestors. Prolonged exposure to stress has a toxic effect on our brain and our body.

We have two biological pathways involved in the stress response:

1. The rapid response autonomic nervous system acts by way of the neurochemicals adrenaline and noradrenalin. This is our fight-or-flight response. The process starts well before we are even aware that a stress alert has been given.
2. The slow-responding hypothalamic-pituitary-adrenal (HPA) axis activates the stress hormone cortisol. This indicates a chronic stress mode. Cortisol is so powerful that it can change our brain. It can be a very destructive hormone that affects our brain and our body.

It is important for our brain health that we build resilience to stress. Here are some practical tips to become calm and reduce stress:

*   Learn to recognize the triggers that set off a stress response when you are not in danger.
*   Reach out to friends and family. Social connections buffer stress.
*   Cultivate optimism and seek out and savor positive emotions.
*   Do something new. Novel, slightly challenging experiences "inoculate" you against future stress.
*   Exercise daily and sleep nightly
*   Cultivate a mindfulness or meditative practice.

I, for one, think that it is great news that we can take some control over our bodies in a way that leads to a healthy brain. All we have to do is exercise, mentally stimulate ourselves, eat right, socialize, sleep well, and manage the stress in our lives. All these lifestyle pieces contribute to a healthy brain. But you cannot pick or choose which ones you are going to do and neglect the others. They each contribute to brain health, but together, they work synergistically, creating optimal results. Alzheimer's is now being referred to as a lifestyle disease. The healthy practices are all geared to give you a strong, high-functioning body that contributes to a strong, high-functioning brain that can work well for you even as you continue to age. Yes, you can change your body, and you can change your brain.

About the Author

Patricia Faust, MGS, is a gerontologist specializing in the issues of brain aging, brain health, brain function, and dementia. She has a master's degree in gerontological studies from Miami University in Oxford, Ohio. Patricia is a certified brain health coach and received a certification in neuroscience and wellness through Dr. Sarah McKay and the Neuroscience Academy.

My Boomer Brain, founded in 2015, is the vehicle that Patricia utilizes to teach, coach, and consult about brain aging, brain health, and brain function. Her newsletter, My Boomer Brain, has international readers from South Africa, Australia, and throughout Europe and Canada.

Patricia's speaking experience spans the spectrum of audiences as she addresses corporate executives on brain function, regional financial professionals on client-diminished capacity, and various senior venues concerning issues around brain aging and brain health.

Email patricia@myboomerbrain.com
Website: www.myboomerbrain.com

CHAPTER 9

BIOHACKING: TAKE CONTROL OF YOUR OWN BIOLOGY

By Chelsea Fournier
Health & Wellness Mentor, Nutrigenomics and Biohacking
Wilmington, North Carolina

Your genetics load the gun. Your lifestyle pulls the trigger.
—Mehmet Oz

In this book about having a successful body, I am going to share my raw journey about what it feels like to have a very unsuccessful body. My story may have facts unique to me, but it is very relatable to many. By sharing my story, I hope to help you relate to one or more of the four ideas I explore:

1. Most of us truly can't imagine how good our bodies and minds can feel.
2. There is nothing shameful about being unwell.
3. Don't wait for a wake-up call to start a journey to better health.
4. Taking control of your own biology is a possibility through biohacking.

I Couldn't Imagine How Good My Body and Mind Could Feel

One definition of "successful" that I appreciate is "having a favorable or desired outcome." Currently, when I think about a favorable or desired outcome for my body, I picture having lots of energy, focus, strength, proper digestion, and mental clarity. But that wasn't always the case.

Less than a decade ago, I would have told you I was healthy, that I was fine. In fact, I was neither of those things. Just as a person with color blindness cannot be certain they are seeing the color blue correctly, someone who is chronically unwell may not be sure they know what it feels like to be healthy.

At the peak of the 2008 crash, I graduated from law school and accepted a job offer from a top law firm in my market. I was ecstatic to go shopping for suits and heels as I stepped into the life of a corporate lawyer at the age of 24. I liked many aspects of my work. I believed I was really good at what I did. However, this season of my life was when everything came to a head, and it became clear that the lifestyle and demands of my work were taxing my body and mind in ways that were unhealthy.

I Was Ashamed of How Unwell I Was, As Though It Were a Personal Failure

At that time, there were two sides of me in relation to my health. The side everyone saw was me bringing in homemade bread and salads for lunch, leaving for a massage break, squeezing in a workout before 6 am, growing my own produce, going on hiking trips, and taking vitamins by the handful. From the outside, it looked like I lived a healthy lifestyle.

And then there was the side that I hid, out of shame. Between the years 2008 and 2013, there are large chunks of my life that I missed out on because I was fighting an uphill battle. I can recall times when:

- I had to ask my HR department to buy me a special lamp and standing desk, so I could work through chronic headaches and joint pain.
- I had to leave my office to go sit in my car in the parking garage, so I could suffer through a panic attack in private.
- I couldn't stay awake past 8:30 pm because of fatigue, but at 2 am I would be wide awake, staring at the ceiling, tossing and turning for the rest of the night.

- I spent two hours in the bathroom violently ill from food allergy reactions, after eating a "safe" salad at a local steakhouse with a client.
- I cried in the dressing room because I was shopping for a new suit … again … after gaining more weight.
- I spent much of one winter on the couch, coughing all night, to the point I was nervous I had broken a rib.
- I had to be carried down a mountain in the dark because a fever hit me out of nowhere, ruining our trip to a hike-in New Year's Eve cabin get-away.
- I had urinary tract infections and yeast infections back to back for six months.
- I had a menstrual cycle that lasted 120 days, with mind-numbing cramps.

None of these were favorable or desirable outcomes from my great job. None of this felt successful. But, at the time, admitting something was deeply wrong was too overwhelming. My poor health felt like a chink in the armor of the successful appearance I wanted to convey.

I powered through these challenges, without slowing down the demands of my life or career. I downplayed how I felt. I was making efforts but getting no results from the diet changes, supplements, or workouts I was trying. I was giving up hope that anything could help me, so I just tried to manage and hide what was going on.

My Wake-Up Call

In March of 2014, I received a phone call that was the catalyst for major change in my life.

I was in Las Vegas for a work conference, just starting to unpack in the hotel, when I saw a number dialing in from my doctor's office. I had finally caved and gone in for some testing right before I left for the trip. My doctor called me personally on a weekend with results. She asked if I had something to take notes with.

She jumped right in, rattling off facts. A diagnosis, an acronym, books I should buy, and a medication I would be on for life. She ended with a very matter-of-fact statement that it would be unlikely I could have children without medication or intervention. She suggested that if having children was a goal of mine, I should start looking into options sooner than later.

I hung up and looked at my notes, a bit dazed and very confused. Through all the notes scratched on the sheet, all I saw was "NO BABY" in caps, circled three times. Despite all the health issues I had been facing and the stress I was under, I had been trying to get pregnant unsuccessfully for two years. It was a huge strain on my already crumbling marriage. The pit in my stomach felt heavy and dark, as my mind spiraled to worst-case scenarios. And I spent the rest of the night at the open bar numbing my fears, until the sun came up.

Later that morning, I nursed my hangover and took out my journal. I began writing all the reasons and ways I could turn this into a positive. I became determined to reclaim my health and make whatever changes were necessary to prove the doctor wrong. I wanted to create a vessel that my future baby would grow healthy and strong in. And without medical intervention.

I finally admitted to myself that I had normalized being chronically sick and had given up on the hope of feeling well. When it was just about me, I could power through it. But I wasn't willing to power through and miss my chance to have the family I had always wanted.

I met with my doctor again when I returned home, and I tried her method of treatment for a total of five days. After feeling horrible side effects and doing my own research on long-term risks, I stopped the medication cold turkey and cancelled my follow-up appointments. I became a voracious researcher and learner, and I began exploring alternative health modalities and lifestyle changes that might benefit me. I advocated for myself and became stubbornly committed to following through with the changes I pursued.

The rest of 2014 and 2015 were a whirlwind in ways I had never even considered. The shorthand version is that in those two years I worked up the courage to strip out everything in my life that caused me more stress than I could handle while healing. I left my failing marriage, and we amicably fast-tracked a divorce. I took a sabbatical from my career, trusting that I could grow my online side hustle into something bigger. I moved in with my sister and took on creating a positive mindset for health and hope like it was a full-time job. I made vision boards, said positive healing affirmations, and read book after book about healing, health, and positivity. At the same time, I was being introduced to the concept of biohacking.

Biohacking Became My Way to Take Back Control

Biohacking was a new term to me. Basically, biohacking is finding ways to take control of your biology. If you've researched and pursued ways to improve your health, you are a biohacker without knowing the label. But biohacking is more than just guessing what changes to make and hoping for a positive result. It is about understanding why you feel, think, and perform certain ways. Biohacking is getting to know your body and learning how to positively tweak how you feel for optimal health and well-being.

We live in a world that is constantly hijacking our bodies and cells in ways we literally can't keep up with. No other generation has had to deal with EMF exposure, toxic products, water pollution, chemical exposure, poor food quality, and the many other stressors that we experience today. Looking back, when I was at my rock bottom, I was eating an alarming amount of sugar, like an addict, consuming alcohol to numb my stress, and doing high intensity workouts that taxed my body in an attempt to lose weight. I was unaware of the ingredients in my food or in the body and household products I used, and I was unaware of the high amounts of emotional stress that I was under in my personal and professional life.

It would have been completely overwhelming to tackle overhauling everything at once. So, as I came to know better, I tried to do better. With small tweaks that started to make a big difference, I started my biohacking journey.

For me, the beginning was all about simple lifestyle changes like drinking filtered water, meditating daily, trying gentler exercise options like yoga and walking, finding my optimal sleep cycle, eating more healthy fats, and trying intermittent fasting. But biohacking really ramped up for me when I learned about "nutrigenomics" and how to support my microbiome.

You don't have to be a scientist to benefit from this nerdy-sounding science. Let's look at two specific examples of what biohacking via nutrigenomics can look like in practice, the science behind it, and lifestyle and product regimens that can get to deeper root causes of poor health.

Biohack Your Body with Nutrigenomics and Reduce Your Toxic Load

Nutrigenomics, broken down in its meaning, is looking at how nutrition and natural formulas can impact our DNA structure and genetic expression. Sounds complicated, right? It is actually beautiful in its simplicity.

This area of science tells us that just because we may have a gene for a certain disease or affliction does not mean that it is our destiny. We know what we put in our mouth directly affects the extent to which certain genes are expressed. And we can reverse harmful expressions, such as for disease genes, and increase positive expressions, such as for making more protective antioxidant enzymes. To me, learning about this felt like a way to flip on and off the right switches for a clean slate.

Through my personal work with natural health providers over the years, I know I have genetic markers that make it incredibly hard for my body to detoxify chemicals and toxins. I'll add that up to 40 percent of the population has similar genetic defects impacting their detoxing abilities. When your cells cannot detox properly, it is as if trash is backing up in your cells—this trash is called free radicals or oxidative stress. Over time, the cells cannot function properly. This can have big consequences in relation to DNA repair, mood regulation, mental health, reproductive health, overall cell function, and how we experience health.

I grew up in the '80s and '90s using fragranced lotions, perfumes, body splashes, chemical hair removers, heavy duty cleaners, and eating without regard to organic labels or ingredients. Even if my body could detox normally, I likely had a high toxic load accrued in my body. Toxic load is a term referring to the accumulation of toxins and chemicals in our body from foods and things we ingest, the water we drink, the personal care products we use, and environmental exposures.

If you are experiencing chronic health issues or just want to feel better, exploring biohacking to intentionally reduce your toxic load is a simple starting point. You can make conscious choices about what you are ingesting and exposing yourself to. I personally no longer buy products with "fragrance" or "parfum" as ingredients, I make sure almost all of my produce and meat purchased is organic, and I am very attentive to ingredients and labels of personal care and cleaning products I use in my home.

I also use a natural nutrigenomic product that is proven to reduce oxidative stress—that trash building up in our cells—by up to 40 percent in 30 days. It also helps the body detoxify genes, keeping the master blueprint of the cell's function intact, and supports the body's natural ability to repair and rejuvenate cells. So, as I know better and do better going forward, this creates a solid foundation for cellular health.

When I began using this one product back in 2013, I very quickly started to notice real benefits in my day-to-day life. I began to sleep better and wake more rested. I began feeling stronger, have more energy, was in a better mood, and began to experience more vitality. And as I began to feel better and have more energy and clarity, I was encouraged to keep going on my health journey and commit to other lifestyle biohacks.

Biohack Your Immune System Function for an Optimal Mood

Ready for a few wild facts about your gut? There are nearly 100 trillion microorganisms in our intestines and microbiome. Our microbiome, in brief, is basically the mix of bacteria and microorganisms living in our gut. Roughly 80 percent of our immune system lives in our gut, and we are learning more about the connection between our gut and our brain / mental health (I encourage you to search "gut-brain axis" online to learn more.) Yet many of us give no thought to how we can keep those microorganisms alive and well, or the impact their health has on how we live and feel.

My prolonged and recurrent illnesses were a cause of concern for me. As were my food allergies, sugar addiction, and mood swings. Much of my research led me to improving my gut health. As I learned more about what can harm our microbiome, I realized I had not been very kind to it over the years. I was a binge drinker from a young age, a sugar addict, and had been on multiple rounds of antibiotics several years in a row. All these factors, along with high stress and high toxic load, can be extremely damaging to the good bacteria that make up a healthy microbiome in the gut.

In 2015, I decided to completely stop drinking alcohol, stop eating processed sugar, and limit my dairy intake for 90 days to see how I felt. I also started finding ways to consume good probiotic foods in my diet such as sauerkraut, pickles, and other fermented foods. I did this to give some love to all those microorganisms. At first, it was incredibly challenging, and label reading became frustrating (sugar is in everything by the way). But five years later, as I write this, it is now just my normal way of living and eating, and I absolutely feel the difference.

I know that supporting my microbiome through food sources is a good start, but I also utilize high-quality probiotic and prebiotic supplements daily to help plant a high amount of good bacteria and make sure they can grow properly in my gut to flourish. This helps to boost my immune system, regulate moods, and decreases incidences of food allergies or cravings.

My Updates as a Biohacking Change-Maker

While I don't believe in before-and-after stories, here's a quick update on what has happened since that call in 2014. I maintain a healthy weight, have more optimal digestion, have a stronger immune system function, and feel younger and stronger now in my late 30's, than I did in my 20's. I am rarely sick, and when I am, I recover very quickly. I am more in tune with how good makes me feel than ever before, and I love cooking health foods for my family.

And a little life update—I never went back to practicing law full-time. I did turn my online side hustle into more, and now I help other families develop home-based businesses as well. My heartache turned to bliss when I met my soulmate. And now I have him as a lifelong biohacking partner, along with our son. We welcomed our sweet baby to the world November 3, 2019, after a natural pregnancy.

I would never claim that any one specific biohack, product, or tweak cured me of anything. But, my work as a biohacker created the vessel my son needed after all, and it's a vessel I am much happier living in.

Biohacking is a movement and is available to everyone. Whether you want to explore free or low-cost lifestyle changes, or invest in science-backed nutrigenomic products or supplements, it's a fascinating area to begin researching and exploring for people of all walks of life. Through biohacking, you can take control over your life. I encourage you to start right now. Pull the trigger and get your life on track.

About the Author

In her late 20s, Chelsea Fournier received a health diagnosis that caused her to overhaul her health and life. Since 2013, she has embraced the life of a bio-hacker, looking for ways to up-level her health, focus, motivation, and energy with lifestyle, nutrition, and product regimens that make her feel amazing. She believes that most people truly don't know how good their bodies are made to feel. She wants to help you find out for yourself.

Chelsea is a (recovering) lawyer, a coach, and a leader in network marketing. She is the lucky mama to the sweetest Baby E, wife to her amazing adventure buddy Bernie, and a biohacker for life.

If you would like to learn how you could start a journey towards more Activated Living, or book time for a free Focus & Power Up Call to get customized suggestions on biohacking steps you can take, please contact her directly. Chelsea would be honored to connect and help you on your journey.

Email: chelsea@chelseafournier.com
Website: www.chelseafournier.com/activated-living

CHAPTER 10
MOHARA: THE FULCRUM OF A WARRIOR

By Rolando Garcia, III
Martial Arts Instructor, Fitness Industry Leader
New York, New York

Love everyone, but never sell your sword.
—Paulo Coelho

I have lived my entire life as a martial artist. My immersive study of the science of martial disciplines has shaped my entire development. My continued evolution as a human being owes much to the path of the traditional warrior and artist. To be clear, this is first and foremost a spiritual undertaking, as it deals with the complex and ultimate matter of life and death in this universe. It is through arduous physical training and conditioning of the body that we penetrate into the spiritual.

I first undertook this path as a child through my father. He shared with me a comprehensive curriculum that included training in Zen, Judo, and Eskrima, among others. Eskrima, a traditional fighting system from the Philippines, quickly introduced me to the harsh reality of weapons-based training of the Eskrimador. Judo introduced me to physical pressure and anatomical leverage. My Zen studies brought me face to face with all that was deep within me. As I hurtle through my humble portion of infinite space and time, it is the martial disciplines that awaken me to the present and the now.

There are serious consequences in individual and mass combat. History can provide us with descriptions of military victory (overwhelmingly or narrowly so), but it is the martial disciplines that teach us to understand the mechanisms and processes of universal conflict. Textbooks relay historical context and desired outcomes; martial disciplines teach a timeless context and prepare us for any and all outcomes. History outlines the consequences of others' actions while studying the martial arts develops in us the ability to carefully weigh our own.

In the matter of immersing yourself in the study of traditional martial weaponry, take great care in your approach to the practice. It takes being humble, with the deepest sincerity and devotion, searching only to refine your physicality and your character, thereby elevating your life. This practice will introduce you to your full capabilities as both a peaceful and warring being, as both aggressor and defender, as both a physical and spiritual being in pursuit of aligning yourself with the truth, through the artistic depth of your practice.

Above all, take this to your heart: in the study of martial weaponry, *the instrument teaches your mind and body* correct movement, correct biomechanics, correct technique, and correct decisions. You will reap the *physical and mental* benefits of this study only when you humble yourself to what the instrument will teach you *about yourself*, thereby giving you insight to all manner of human movement, thinking, and decision-making.

On the Matter of Dizon

Felicissimo Dizon, a formidable and enigmatic Eskrimador, a discerning instructor, and incomparable Filipino death-match master, codified an art he named "Mohara." As relayed to my father (at the time, Dizon's private student and a young attorney in his 20s), Dizon felt the art of Mohara was his "ultimate" expression and understanding of personal combat. He taught my father several curriculums—all of which led to his prized Mohara, which he deemed the most difficult to master. He shared the art with my father, who then taught the curriculum of techniques and methodologies to me, only after several decades of intense study and training.

For background, death-matches in the Philippines were common in the early and mid-20th century. Both un-armored practitioners often chose sticks of varying lengths as their weapons of choice. These were often no-holds-barred affairs, similar to today's MMA events, but without the rules. In the case of

Filipino death-matches, fast-moving sticks (often invisible to the eye) add an exponential complexity—unexpected angles, false leads, reduced margin of error, unconventional footwork, and an inner reckoning of one's willingness to engage. Even the most glancing of blows would lead to devastating injuries (specifically to joints); direct blows to certain parts of the anatomy along the midline would often result in death. As a reminder—only a few years earlier Filipino Eskrimadors fought openly on the battlefield with the more well-armed Spaniards, then the US Marines, and only a few short years later were deep in the mountains, fighting a guerilla war against the occupying Imperial Japanese Army. Sport and combat achieve their definitions depending on an arbitrary historical timeline. For us, such matches serve no purpose and become fodder for internet discussions. For those who lived through the horrors of WWII in the Philippines, the matter of death matches only needed a nod of resolution—it was not up for discussion.

Dizon, in this timeline and unforgiving environment, was considered unmatched and without peer. Through relatives, mutual friends, and students, stories were relayed to my father about his soft-spoken and stoic master; stories that the man was simply too humble to convey himself. All the descriptions aligned: he was indomitable, powerful even in stride, pure in his devotion to his definition of the art, and simply in a class unto himself. Dizon went for years without a single defeat, without declining a single match. He taught only a handful of students. Some observed that his criteria for selection placed an extraordinary emphasis on character and temperament over skill and physical prowess. Some also observed that he preferred mostly to train alone in the deep mountains, rumored to be sinister and haunted. He would return, only several days later.

Death-matches were not always ringside events. Sometimes they started with a simple request for a "light" sparring match in a casual setting such as behind a street-side food stand during lunch, or on an empty patch of provincial land while traveling. Dizon would acquiesce to such requests, even in the middle of lunch, accompanying the challenger behind a building, only to come back a few moments later with the challenger vanquished. He would finish his meal as if nothing had happened.

My father met Dizon when the master was in his late 50s. What stands out to my father's mind when training with Dizon was his powerful physique despite being middle-aged. Stocky with broad shoulders and muscular arms, he stood with an elegant posture and a stoic manner, with a full head of dark hair. His movements were smooth, as he seemed to glide with minimal effort, often leaving my father shocked with how easily he positioned himself outside of my father's peripheral vision during sparring matches. As my father tried to grasp what had just happened, he would sense a tapping on his neck or shoulder with the unmistakable rattan stick of his teacher.

"How did I end up here? And how did you end up there?" he would ask my father. "Buhos at buhos," he would say, the English translation being "to pour it on." During his death-matches, he would glide into position behind his opponent (out of his line of sight), upon which time he would rain full power strikes to end the match decisively. It is said that the technique became his signature finish, which led to his years of dominance. As my father progressed in training, he shared an even clearer and all-encompassing vision of victory:

> "To win at all costs is easy, but it should not be our aim. Our aim
> is to win in such a manner that the very heart of who you are is
> revealed in your victory. That is what Mohara demands."

Mohara and the Complexity of Movement

Dizon created Mohara as an attempt to decode the requirements of a more complex and volatile time. Violence could, and often would, erupt from three specific sources, and usually without notice: the casual challenge, the death match in front of a wild audience, or mass warfare. To live in a time where just one of these factors was to be prevalent would make for complex social interaction indeed. To imagine that a substantial stretch of history involved the very real existence of all three boggles the mind. The degree of violence is further complicated by the seeming quantum nature of its appearance–without warning and without notice, one's physical body, one's life, is either interrupted or ended, seemingly without cause or a fluid narrative.

Dizon's Mohara, with its emphasis on twisting footwork, mental and physical agility, strong yet interchangeable grips, spells out the requirements clearly to its devotees—the matter of becoming a warrior requires a deep and constant commitment to physical, mental, and spiritual sharpening. To run mindlessly forward or backward (as one would on a treadmill), would be a poor strategy to implement when faced with someone who is armed and skilled. To lift or brace (as one would with a bench press) would also be suboptimal, as it does not prime our neural responses for the onslaught of feedback that comes from such a sensory-rich environment (again, your armed and skilled opponent).

Although there are many great benefits to be found in popular exercise routines accompanied by music, mirrors, and other attention grabbers, in Mohara training, there is no checking a mobile device during training, no TV, no loud music, no colored lights, no group to hide in—no opportunity to check out and simply become unaware of yourself and your surroundings. In Mohara, you are *holding a traditional weapon*, clearly spelling out your responsibility to your training, to your devotion to your well-being as well as that of others, and your absolute focus on and respect for your instructor who, in the words of Dizon, "paid the price of this knowledge by risking *his life*." To receive such instruction, in this day and age, demands more than a monthly membership and regular attendance to become worthy of being its recipient. It requires a reckoning with one's character, devotion, personal integrity, purpose, and overall place in the world.

As such, the progression of training in Mohara can be divided into three categories

- Flow
- Strategy
- Power

On Flow: "How Did I End Up Here?"

Flowing with a 36-inch stick is the first consideration of Mohara for several reasons. Firstly, since the art focuses on handling the stick with one hand, familiarity with the instrument, under varying conditions, is the first goal. Familiarity with the stick means being able to move one's body fluidly in a coordinated and uninterrupted manner. Traditional Eskrima recommends a shorter stick between 24 and 28 inches, for practical purposes. (As Dizon once told my dad, "If you're able to find a stick of your favored length in a fight, you're a lucky man indeed.") So, why the 36-inch stick? Simple. It presents a unique challenge to the practitioner (as a reminder, Mohara is the advanced curriculum to his overall system) by increasing the likelihood of unwittingly hitting your surroundings (your ceiling, furniture, chairs, the ground), other people (family members, roommates, oblivious pets), or yourself (your opposing arm, your legs, your head) with your own stick.

The margin for error, in Mohara, is narrower than in other curriculums. As mentioned earlier, Mohara leaves no opportunity to mentally check out.

Secondly, flowing with a 36-inch stick in a single-handed manner requires a constant, inward focus with a *concurrent* spatial awareness. Proper biomechanics, hyper awareness of footwork (placement, weight distribution, and sequence), breathing apparatus, energy conservation, total integration, and thought awareness and management—these are all integral to developing and maintaining a flow between offense, defense, and countering techniques. Moving in unison *with* the stick is an entirely different matter than simply moving *the* stick. The flow of your own body and the stick become one synchronized movement.

As a result of this practice, flowing in Mohara leads to the mind-state required to accept any and all challenges: a state of calm and *instinctive* resolution where the body and mind deeply become one. One of Dizon's nicknames was "Dizon All-the-Time," which meant that he accepted all challengers and challenges. As one would flow in practice, one would flow with the challenges of life and, perhaps, in anticipating it, shock the challenger into disarray.

On Strategy: "How Did You End Up There?"

Strategy becomes the emergent focus of the practitioner once there is an acceptable calm flow in training. The introduction of a similarly flowing, but *uncooperative* partner, is now introduced. At the level of Mohara, unlike traditional Eskrima, there are no fixed drills or partner drills. At the level that Dizon required, Mohara is meant to make the practitioner more intuitive and more reliant on an inward determination. Positioning, angling, and countering all become matters of practical and creative problem-solving that appear in the moment but are not fixed in a curriculum. The process of developing strategy is an individual and organic determination, but the conclusions almost often remain the same. You have out-positioned and out-struck your opponent while all his resources have been directed to a ghost-like target that no longer exists in space and time. (As a side-note: I believe that, in the end, masters like Dizon frequented the haunted mountains of the Philippines to achieve a similar outcome. He was studying the nature and strategy of "ghosts").

As such, the introduction of an uncooperative partner is not only a technical challenge similar to a sparring match, but a challenge to the practitioner's ability to maintain an internal equilibrium while you present a challenge to disrupt your partner's. That is the strategic goal of Mohara.

On Power: "Buhos at Buhos"

From a practical standpoint, once proficiency in flow and strategy are achieved, the final piece of the Mohara puzzle is to develop power as a unified expression of one's *entire* being. Flow develops uninterrupted movement, strategy develops quantum decision-making in the face of resistance, and power develops one's resolve. It is important in Mohara for every moment and decision to embody the power of the individual executing it. There are martial arts styles that seek an exceptional reliance on technique alone while quelling personal expression and the spirit of the practitioner. Perhaps the conditions of the fog of war require this approach. In Mohara, the goal is to subsume the individual so that they are indistinguishable from the art itself. It is in the end, the realization of a warrior ideal—the art is inseparable from the artist—the body inseparable from the system.

From the perspective of force production, the body and the stick are one. What was once an unwieldy encumbrance that seemed to move of its own accord has become—through lengthy and devoted practice—a trusted companion. As such, the practitioner will move with greater ease and deliberation, and come to rely on his art in all matters. What was once a grand effort by the arm and wrist has become the subtle and more integrated movement of a more powerful fulcrum—the hips, feet, and a grounded center (part of why I believe Dizon moved with such grace and subtlety). As such, Mohara became the pinnacle and most complex achievement of Dizon's artistry because, in the simplest terms, *he shifted the fulcrum of the art*. When his finishing blows rained upon his opponents, it was not the stick alone nor a well-trained technician that struck. Dizon came upon them with the full weight and expression of his entire being. Thus, the heart of the warrior is revealed.

Blaze Like Meteors

My lifelong devotion to martial arts training has promoted a daily deepening of my understanding, respect, and discipline within myself. Eskrima gave me something to respect. At first it was respect for a martial instrument, and what secret forces lay dormant within it. That respect then extended to others' skills and perspectives. As my own power emerged through my physical and mental refinement, I came to realize that the art had been teaching me how to respect myself completely. To paraphrase 13th century Zen Master Dōgen regarding intimate oneness, "Moment by moment a thought appears and disappears without abiding. Moment by moment a body appears and disappears without abiding. Yet the power of practice always matures."

Eskrima allowed me to first understand myself within the art through constant physical and mental preparation. It allowed me to face personal, professional, and spiritual challenges as opportunities to mature, develop, and overcome. Dizon's Mohara led me to arrive, ultimately, to the deepest point of the journey—finding the art within myself.

The purpose of warriorship—and perhaps all physical training—is to deepen and unite every facet of the body and mind to dwell under the will of the practitioner, and to instantly reveal the truth of one's being. All athletic feats and challenge events are measures of this heroic evidence of willful causality, in a universe where the fates of all beings, including those of blazing meteors and massive stars, are determined seemingly without order or care.

When an athlete throws a shot-put, we consider the distance a spectacular feat not because of its objective measure, but because we see a unification of mental focus and physical force under the willful command of an individual that the immortal stars are seemingly indifferent toward. What is a javelin throw or a 100-meter sprint compared to the speed at which our tiny planet traverses through space? What is the mass of Betelgeuse which is 1,000 times the mass of our own sun compared to the immeasurable will of a sentient, upright human being who *connects* to a force from within? No matter how diminutive in scale, our human ability to focus the body and mind can be compared to a vastly more forceful yet unscripted universe.

The Eskrimador may appear sporadically in matches throughout his short life, even enlist in full-scale warfare that will be recorded in the pages of books. However, it is only the most devoted who believe that the way can be found daily in the infinite spaces of the heart. Within the heart, we can decode all our movements. Our practice brings us deeper to this point, with each stroke and shift. However subtle and imperceptible, this process occurs without abiding.

We will all, in our own time, be interrupted by an upstart challenger, or perhaps proceed through a darkness that beckons to us like a haunted forest. We may be forced to answer in our own way how we got from one moment and how we plan to get to the next. What trusted companions we have at the time certainly matter, but what is more important is the art we carry within, so that we may resolve the matter simply, with a nod toward the unknown. This art has been within us before the beginning and will stay with us far into that good night. For Dizon, my father, and myself, the name of that art is Mohara. It is the fulcrum of a warrior.

About the Author

Rolando Garcia, III is an experienced leader and manager in sales, operations, and P&L optimization in the luxury health, fitness, and wellness space. Featured in *Forbes*, the *New York Post*, and *Self Magazine*, Rolando has worked in leadership roles at world renowned organizations such as Equinox (as the general manager of the award-winning elite, private, and luxurious E at Columbus Circle in NYC), LifeTime (as GMIT of Manhattan's luxurious Life Time Sky), and Orangetheory. He is currently the NYC regional manager for Corporate-Owned Studios at Orangetheory.

Rolando holds a master's certificate in Service and Hospitality at Cornell University's School of Hotel Administration. He is a member of Mensa International, the high-IQ society that accepts only the top 2% of its applicants. Classically trained in Shakespeare, he completed his studies at NYC's National Shakespeare Conservatory.

Rolando is the author of Intrinsic *Excellence: Business Development and Leadership Systems for Success in Personal Training* (Dragondoor Publications, 2016), and he is a public speaker on health, fitness, wellness, and performance management. As an accomplished martial artist, Rolando is a Certified Full Instructor in Jeet Kune Do/Filipino Martial Arts, along with additional instructor credentials in Boxe Francaise Savate and Brazilian Jiu-Jitsu. He is also an RKC Level II Instructor in Russian Kettlebells and a Precision Nutrition Level II Coach. He was an active amateur competitor in Brazilian Jiu Jitsu, Muay Thai, and Filipino Stick Fighting. Upon retiring in 2005, he opened his own academy in Manhattan, which at the time housed the only Savate Curriculum in NYC.

The focus of Rolando's training remains his beloved Eskrima and Dizon's Mohara. He is currently studying traditional Japanese Swordsmanship, with a focus on Shinkage-Ryu Hyoho. He resides in New Jersey with his wife, Michelle, and his two cats, Mary Ellen and Tesshū, named after the 19th century samurai, poet, and calligraphist, Yamaoka Tesshū.

Email: RolandoGarcia3iii@gmail.com
LinkedIn: https://www.linkedin.com/in/rolando-garcia-iii-48341715/

CHAPTER 11
THE FITNESS MINDSET

By Roy E. Hatcher
Fitness and Wellness Coach, Advocate for Toxin-Free Living
Henderson, Nevada

Whether you think you can, or think you can't, either way you're right.
—Henry Ford

Henry Ford's famous quote is so true because your success in anything is all about your mindset and your attitude. Your attitude is a huge factor in determining your success or failure in all aspects of your life.

The Google dictionary definition of fitness is "The condition of being physically fit and healthy." Many don't realize that *disease* and *lack of fitness* are closely related. The goal of this chapter is not to have you become a fitness fanatic, but rather to open your eyes and your mind to the benefits of healthy living and fitness. A **fitness mindset** will keep you moving forward and making daily progress in your efforts to lose weight, get in shape, be fit, and live a healthier lifestyle.

When you begin to think about fitness and working out, your mind will most likely object. You will be able to come up with all kinds of excuses and reasons to justify why you should not become fit. Often people complain about the expense of joining a gym, or the time it takes to go workout when they are already time poor. I've got news for you—the time is never right, so you have to start now.

There are many solutions to overcoming the challenge of time, and one of those solutions is just changing your mindset. Your mindset should be "I MUST START NOW." It is also important to start where you are and make daily changes to improve your overall health and lifestyle. Your mindset can impact failure or success. Your beliefs, whether good or bad, play a pivotal role in whether you achieve your goal. Your beliefs also play a critical role on how you deal with everyday challenges in life. STOP PROCRASTINATING and START TODAY.

What is **mindset**? The definition of mindset is "The established set of attitudes held by someone." Mindset is the window through which you see yourself. What are YOUR attitudes? Here are examples of some common "fixed" attitudes that could hinder us from accomplishing of our goals:

1. It's too late to start now.
2. I take feedback as a personal attack.
3. I always struggle with …
4. Either I'm good at something, or I'm not.
5. There's no point in trying if I'm just going to fail.

Now look at these same attitudes with a different mindset:

1. I can learn whatever I want or need to learn.
2. I can find value in every bit of feedback I receive.
3. I can always do better at something if I want to, but it will take some effort.
4. If I'm not good at something, I can become better at it through practice.
5. I see failure as an opportunity to learn, reassess, and do a better next time.

Please allow me to share my story with you. I believe that it will give hope to the hopeless and help you on your journey to a successful body.

I was 32 years old when I got my "desk" job with the State of Michigan. I had a daily routine of stopping for coffee and doughnuts on the way to work. I LOVE doughnuts! I always made it a point to get two doughnuts because one was never enough, and besides, they tasted so good. Every day, my lunch consisted of a Big Mac and fries with iced tea. In less than four months, I had enlarged my waist by five inches. I remember getting out of the shower one day, and when I stepped in front of the mirror, I said, "Yikes! Who is that guy?"

A quick self-diagnosis told me that I had "Dunlap Disease." That is where your belly has done lapped over your belt! The prognosis was heart attack, diabetes, high blood pressure, cholesterol issues, shortness of breath, lack of motivation, and a host of other things. I knew that I didn't like the way I looked, I didn't like the way I felt, and I didn't like the extra weight. And I didn't like myself! I knew then that I needed to make a change but wasn't sure where to start.

Some of my friends suggested running, others suggested diets. Many said it is part of getting old. Others were adamant that my condition was "normal" and would only get worse as I approached forty years old. I didn't like what I was hearing, so I decided to check out a gym that was offering a 30-day trial membership with classes. And, I joined.

I was not an ideal student at the gym, especially at the start, but I kept with it, and I learned how to keep going, how to push my body, and how to reach goals. As I reflect on my experience, I realize that there were a few things that worked for me, and these might also work for your journey to a successful body too. Here are five key rules:

RULE #1: Start Now! Start Today!

Day one was a Monday, and all day at work I dreaded the thought of going to the gym. My brain was coming up with all the excuses why I should not go. Reluctantly, after work, I rushed to the gym. I wanted to be early, so I could sit in my car and watch who was coming in and going out of the gym. I saw sculpted women and rock-solid men, thin waistlines, big pumped chests, massive arms, and absolutely nobody that looked like me.

As I sat there, FEAR started to creep in, and I knew, at that very moment, I had two choices: Fear Everything And Run or Face Everything And Rise. I chose Face Everything And Rise! Why? Because I remembered a friend telling me that option one, once chosen, will be chosen almost as a default throughout the rest of my life.

I jumped out of the car and ran to the front door before I could hear my inner voice tell me to leave again. The people at the gym welcomed me and told me I would be in the class on the right. I walked into the room and to my surprise there were only two guys in this class … Fred and me. What a shock.

Immediately, my mind was flooded with all the negative thoughts and the mindset, "This isn't for me." My inner voice shouted at me to leave now, but my gut said to stay. And then more people arrived.

After completing that class, which was more of a Zumba-type workout, I went straight to the front desk and inquired about the class. I told them that they must have put me in the wrong class. I asked my trainer, "Why did you put me in that class with all those ladies and no weights? I am here to build some muscle and lose some weight!"

My trainer solemnly looked at me and asked, "How did you like the class?"

I responded, "It was alright, but I thought we would be doing weight training."

He then asked a second question, "Were you able to complete the exercises at all the stations?"

My response to that question was a very quick, "No, not all of them."

RULE #2: We All Have to Start Somewhere

My trainer then proceeded to tell me, "Sir, it seems like your body weight is all the weight you needed to start with for now."

I was furious! On my drive home, I had to reflect on the truth of his words, and I knew he was right, so I stuck with it. I completed the 30-day training and signed a one-year membership contract. I started with free weights, 20 pounds, 30 pounds, 40 pounds, and continued to see improvement in "that guy" in the mirror.

Seven months later someone at the gym asked me to become a trainer. I had shed the weight and lost 6.5 inches from my waistline. I attended the gym five to six days a week, focusing on my weakest areas. I was *consistent* and strived daily to get better. After some time, I became a personal trainer and started training others in the evenings. This gave me a "why" that really kept me motivated. I had to show up because there were people counting on me to help them and encourage them.

My advice to you then is to find someone who is trying to accomplish the same or similar goals as you and partner with them. This works well for encouragement because you will be empathetic towards them, and you can encourage and empower one another. Remember to treat yourself like someone you are responsible for helping; this will help you to consider what would truly be good for you as you help others.

RULE #3: Create Good Habits and Set Goals

Setting goals is an excellent start to creating good habits. These behaviors, whether positive or negative, typically take about 21 days to evolve and become habits. By becoming consistent with our habits, we can achieve goals that we thought were insurmountable. The accomplishment of these goals as part of your daily lifestyle will not only give you *confidence*, but will allow you to set larger, long-term goals, and be successful at achieving them.

Start by setting small goals. When a goal is achieved, it's a great time to reward yourself for completing that goal. These goals can be daily, weekly, and monthly goals. These goals can also be set hourly for those who struggle in the area of excess weight. Here is an example: I am *not* going to eat a candy bar, but instead I will eat a handful of nuts. I am *not* going to have a doughnut, but instead I will eat fruit. I am *not* going to drink a soda, but instead I am going to have a smoothie. I am *not* going to smoke a cigarette, but instead I am going to do ten pushups.

If you have been working on a goal to get rid of excess weight, and you think of searching for food in your kitchen at night, it is not willpower that will prevent you from eating a bowl of food. It is the *habit* of self-control and discipline that will ensure that you don't break your diet plan or deviate from your goals. Learn to replace the negative habit with a positive, uplifting, make-you-feel-better habit. Your attempts at controlling your mental state and your negative thoughts will be futile without good habits to affirm and control your mindset.

To create a fitness or healthier mindset, start with what I call a REPLACEMENT ROUTINE. This is where you replace a negative thought or habit with a positive mantra or habit. For example: on my one-hour lunch break, I picked up fast food, ate, and scrolled social media. I replaced this with a positive habit, which was walking 20 minutes, eating healthy leftovers from dinner, or a healthy lunch for 20 minutes, then another 20 minutes to walk back to work. Right now, many of you likely had the following negative thought, "What if I only have 30 minutes?" The answer: walk ten minutes, eat ten minutes, walk another ten minutes. A healthy lifestyle does not mean deprivation, but discipline and consistency. Discipline is a key factor when it comes to changing your mindset.

RULE #4: Your Only Competition Is You

The only person you are in competition with is the person in the mirror and that is *you*! Do *not* start comparing yourself to others, the skinny or buff guy or gal at the gym. Compare yourself only to who you were yesterday, *not* to who someone else is today!

Good things require work, but merely thinking about a task is not enough to get it done. The weights won't lift themselves. The book won't read itself. You need to put in the effort, the work. You *must* take action.

Start your action by creating positive thoughts. Then dwell on these positive thoughts. Create a mental picture of what you want to look like or what you would like your eating plan to look like. Picture yourself with a pumped chest or a slim waistline, and see how good that makes you feel.

Your mind can trick you into believing a lie if you don't "intentionally" try to build up a resistance to that lie through positive thoughts and affirmations. The key to fighting off this false information is knowledge. Rather than jumping to conclusions, seek knowledge, so it is easier to overcome that negative thought or premonition, like those prejudiced and biased ideas and comments that your so-called friends will be sure to point out to you.

The mind and body cannot operate independent of each other. If you ignore one or the other, they will both malfunction. These two, body and mind, must be controlled as a unit since one affects the other. They depend on one another to thrive, and they must be taken care of simultaneously for best and lasting results.

RULE # 5: Keep a Scorecard

It is imperative that you keep track of your met and unmet goals. Your accomplished goals should be rewarded, and your unmet goals should be reviewed. A new game plan should be set up, put in place, and a start date attached to that plan to accomplish unmet goals. Remember, a goal without a date is just a wish. Keep a scoreboard of how many times you go to the gym. How many times did you run, do pushups, walk, eat healthy, read a chapter in a book, and encourage other people? Keep track of it all because this will help you continually see your results as well as see areas in which you need to put more energy. You will find motivation in simply seeing the number of small or large things you've accomplished as you work toward your successful body.

Here is the takeaway. One doughnut did not make me overweight. One doughnut twice a day, 20 days a month, for four months caused my weight problem. If you do the math that was 160 donuts in four months. I would not have had a weight problem if I had disciplined myself to one doughnut a week or two doughnuts a month. It was my habit that had to change.

The right daily habits over time lead to *big results* and SUCCESS! Do not overthink or complicate this. YOUR successful body is on the way. *Never quit* and *never give up!* Your *best you* is yet to come. You got this.

About the Author

Roy Hatcher is an advocate for toxin-free living as well as a fitness and wellness coach at RNB Health. He grew up in Detroit, Michigan, graduated high school in three years, and continued his education at several different colleges/universities. He has numerous associate degrees, as well as a bachelor's degree in sociology/political science, and a "PhD" in Life! Roy is never afraid of challenges and hard work, and he lives by the biblical statement, I can do all things through Christ who strengthens me (Philippians 4:13).

On top of his work in fitness, Roy has traveled to numerous places around the world and has lived in many of the 50 states. He served his country in the US Army, which also gave him the opportunity to live in Europe. He continues to pursue an adventurous lifestyle and has a passion for helping others to discover their best health through fitness and toxin-free living.

Roy's hobbies consist of motorcycling, golf, reading, and an insatiable appetite for continuous learning. His desire to travel comes from the passion of learning about other cultures and lifestyles. Roy attributes his success to God, his family, and learning to balance the challenges of everyday life. He currently resides in Henderson, Nevada, with his wife, Brenda.

Email: roy@rnbhealth.com
Website: www.rnbhealth.com
LinkedIn: https://www.linkedin.com/in/roy-hatcher-6a419896/

CHAPTER 12

HOT YOGA

By Sarah Jones
Founder of Fierce Bodhi, Yoga Instructor, Encourager
New York Metropolitan Area

A diamond is a chunk of coal that did really well under pressure
—Henry Kissinger

I'd come home late the night before, and there I was, the following morning, back in a place where I didn't want to be. I was trapped in a location where the walls were caving in on me. The department was my cell block, the cubicle was my prison cell, and my manager was the wicked warden. The feeling of being mentally drained was real, and the physical aspect of having to work within a set number of hours, sitting in a cubicle, and staring at a computer confirmed its reality. Not to mention, I noticed that my knees and lower back would stiffen once I got up to use the printer or to meet with co-workers. There was tension in my shoulders and neck causing frequent headaches and discomfort in my upper body. The corporate culture was taking a toll on my body at an early age. Despite all of this, something in the back of my mind just wouldn't let the corporate world be my demise. Welcome to my story of pressure, demands, and unending stress within the corporate culture and how hot yoga was the light that changed my path.

Yoga is an old discipline from India that is both spiritual and physical. It uses breathing techniques, exercise, and meditation to help improve overall health and well-being. My first encounter with yoga came one particular day after work, when I hopped off the train and noticed that a new hot yoga studio was opening directly across the street from my train stop. Being curious, I signed up for a class. After experiencing my first yoga class, it felt like I had drunk euphoria straight out of a glass.

Fast forward a couple of months, and I was lying on my couch feeling a bit under the weather. I was recovering from a bad cold. A sudden onset of a continuous cough attack that felt like I was about to expel a lung. The last cough in the series caused me to throw out my back. Aside from childbirth, it was the most excruciating pain I have ever experienced. I visited a chiropractor, and X-rays revealed that I had a misaligned pelvis by a fraction of an inch, which may have been there from birth. The long, hard cough threw out a disc in my back. The chiropractor's diagnosis: weekly adjustments, walking for an hour each day, and continued practice of hot yoga.

These chiropractic instructions helped me to realign my spine. The entire ordeal had been a blessing in disguise that led me to discover a new lifestyle, embrace the passion of yoga, and eventually teach and inspire all around the world. All I wanted to do was run to my hot yoga classes and let go of everything that didn't serve me throughout my corporate day.

One of my favorite poses is "ragdoll," also known as baddha hasta uttanasana. This is a forward bend at the hips, and the upper body dangles with absolutely no tension while you grasp opposite elbows. It is a simple move often practiced in the beginning sequences of yoga classes in order to find release of stress and promote relaxation in the body.

When I first began yoga, I attended for the relief of stress, and I felt brandnew each time. Little did I know I would soon discover a world of benefits to each pose and would learn of the philosophical advantages as well. Power hot yoga after a day in the corporate compression chamber worked wonders. I practiced the sort of yoga called vinyasa, a series of flowing postures combined with a breath on each movement of the body in a room heated to a temperature of between 95 and 100 degrees.

Best described as a "sweaty hot mess," yoga class left me feeling like I had dropped a load off my shoulders and shed a skin of negativity. I sweated out toxins from the body, such as heavy metals, salt, and, of course, water. Yoga means to "yolk" or to "marry" the breath with the movement, thus becoming one. The heat provides a suppleness to the muscles of the body that allows you to achieve a greater range of motion and ability to stretch further. When performing such rigorous transitional poses, it reduces the risk of injury. This is an important benefit for all people who perform many daily tasks. Also, the high heat puts stress on the cardiovascular system, and the body uses more oxygen, thus creating positive results.

With the proper use of pranayama, controlled breathing techniques, the respiratory system becomes stronger, inducing greater lung capacity. Prana, which is breath, the life-giving force, begins to flow more freely pushing through any emotional and physical blockages, therefore, freeing the body and mind.

Within the first year of practicing, I had my father sign up for a month of yoga on a special deal that the studio was offering. I didn't really think he would come to class; I just wanted the deal. The deal was that if I brought someone who had never attended the studio, we would both receive 50% off the monthly price.

At the time my father joined the yoga studio, he was encountering arthritis in his fingers and his knees, which often bothered him. He decided to take a class, and after taking several classes, he no longer had arthritis in his hands, and the uncomfortable feeling in his knees was reduced. The heat and postural movement increased joint fluid flow, which loosened his stiff joints and decreased the inflammation. Because he saw the results firsthand, my father is an avid yoga practitioner to this day.

Once I found yoga, it became easier for me to go to work every day, but as I was evolving, it was harder to thrive in the corporate culture because my mindset and my priorities were shifting. In many cases, when we engage with the corporate culture, there are social restrictions within the workplace as well as health restrictions in terms of moving around and exercising. For example, in my case, I was forced to sit all day, which is extremely detrimental to a person's health. Several effects include back and spinal injuries, slower metabolism, and chronic pain, just to name a few. And, I know because I experienced these, as have many others in corporate jobs with whom I've spoken.

The great thing about my power hot yoga class was that it countered all the negative effects of my sitting all day. With poses named cat/cow, upward facing dog, ragdoll, seated half-spinal twist, and child's pose, my body was being released from the stillness of my workday. These poses articulate the spine and open space between each vertebra, which results in lengthening the spine rather than compression from a sedentary lifestyle. There is also better circulation of spinal fluid and electrical impulses. The spine is the basis of our bodily structure; a strong spine equals a strong upright body.

Some of the positive effects are not even physical, but mental. Interaction limited to communication over the internet can cause a decline in social involvement and psychological well-being. Also, when the computer is used as the single form of communication, the size of a person's social circle is believed to decline, and feelings of depression and loneliness can increase.

When my father and I joined the yoga studio, not only did we feel different from the classes, but we also felt a sense of belonging to a community. We met new people and became friends within a place that felt sanctimonious. It was a comforting place where everyone knew our names. Not only was there the physical benefit, but we strengthened our bond as we practiced together as father and daughter. We began to share fun experiences at the studio, meet new people, and deepen our trust with each other.

Meanwhile, back at the office, the daily torture of work worsened. Problems arose within my department, and not long afterward, my manager changed their attitude towards me. As a result, I started to worry about getting fired and losing my job. A feeling of inferiority began to settle in my psyche. Every day, there was this heavy weight on my shoulders when I thought about how to deal with my problem. I was so stressed out that I often woke up with anxiety. My face started to break out in hives. There was no amount of makeup that could hide what I was going through. I went to yoga for relief, but for this situation, it only worked temporarily because I knew I had to deal with my work again the following day.

Thank the Lord I was able to land a new position after eight weeks of stress. It was a relief to finally escape that jail cell of a job. But my corporate job wasn't my only stressor in life. My marriage was also so difficult that it was called off by yours truly. This unraveled into a cesspool of guilt and shame during the separation period from my husband. Let me backtrack a bit to explain me and my marriage more.

In my teens and 20s, life was fun. It was easy-breezy throughout high school and college, but then everything started to change. I met someone towards the end of my college years, and little did I know that this someone would be my husband. Even after graduation, I still couldn't decide on what to do with my life. But when he proposed, I figured I would give it a shot. In hindsight, I thought marriage was the right thing to do and the next logical step. It was the example that my parents had given me.

My parents have always been an admirable couple, and I wanted my life to resemble theirs: well put-together, great with kids, yearly anniversaries, and true love. But things just didn't seem to work out that way for me. There was a small still voice in my head that questioned what I was doing with myself. I was a bohemian-spirited girl who wanted to try every adventure and yet ended up in a premature, serious relationship, which led to marriage. Nonetheless, the open-minded me decided to stick it out and see if it could work. So, we stuck it out. We had a child and lived next to my parents, who practically raised my son. Life was grand on the outside; but on the inside, a part of my free spirit had died. I decided to bury it—well, I tried. The desire to let my spirit come alive again just wouldn't leave me alone. Six years into the marriage, I finally chose to strive for my own truth and call it quits. I needed to find myself again.

And, there I was—divorced, with a son, and with no regrets. To this day, I still have a caring relationship with the father of my son, and out of our marriage, we share a beautiful child. It is better I left for my son's sake because he would have gotten the old me instead of the new me, which is a person focused on keeping both my mind and body as healthy as possible.

I knew there was a greater calling in my life, and I didn't know that part of my calling would be helping other corporate employees just like me via yoga. Yoga teaches us to go within ourselves, something called purusha, the eternal authentic spirit. To understand and know the Higher Being within, uncovering the depths of who we are and what we were meant to be and do. I realized that I was solely depending on the physical benefits of yoga to relieve my pain and discomfort in life. However, that is when I learned that yoga offers this benefit of purusha.

For certain instances, it is not enough to attend yoga for the challenging workouts in order to have a successful body. Yoga postures help to eliminate toxic build up in our bodies from stressful negative thinking signifying direct correlation between thought and body. We must learn to discover the root of our issues, where they stem from, and work through them to ultimately free ourselves. Pema Chodron, author of *Wisdom of No Escape*, says, "We learn to acknowledge, embrace, and let go." For many, the perception of yoga is all about downward facing dog, tree pose, and endless chaturangas. But, in yoga, there is also a precious benefit of discovering oneself if one so chooses.

As a little girl, my mother taught me how to pray and be thankful to this "Man upstairs" each night before bed. As I attended Catholic school for all my elementary years, I was again introduced to this Man through ancient biblical stories, teachings from the school nuns, and by attending mandatory Mass every Wednesday. But, as I got older, journeying through high school and college, my church attendance decreased. It wasn't until later as I was going through my separation that a co-worker gave me a message from the Man upstairs. She asked me to attend a non-denominational church with her.

I agreed because I love trying new things and seeing new places. But once I attended, my life took a huge turn. Drowning in guilt, trying to find my way, the random invite allowed me to finally not only meet this Man upstairs, but to begin a journey that was spiritual. This parallel learning of spirituality through the church and yoga made an amazing impression on my life. For many years, I looked at religion as only an organization that instructs the dos and don'ts of life, and if I mess up, then I am a bad person. But according to lessons taught directly from the Bible, there was no way that I would always be perfect.

When practicing in my hot yoga classes, the teacher praised the students that fell out of their poses more than the advanced practitioners that performed the poses perfectly. On quite a few occasions, the teachers taught me about the "process." I learned how to experience the fun in falling and to laugh and not be perfect. Those moments were where the beauty occurred and where growth happened along my journey in yoga, and in my life too.

After several church sermons and hot yoga classes, my guilt and shame began to subside. Prayer life, and my relationship with Jesus, became important to me, and at the same time, yoga taught me the significance of meditation. At the beginning of my hot yoga classes, the teacher always suggested that we set an intention for class, such as peace for someone in a difficult situation, sending love to a family member, or simply showing gratitude. She wanted us to carry this thought for class much like asking or giving thanks, similar to a prayer.

Bible teachings encourage us to meditate on God's word day and night. For me and my life, there was direct correlation between the Bible and yoga. I began to discover more about who I was—a powerful spiritual being, a woman of prayer expanding and rising in love and revelation of my purpose and what I was called to do. No longer did I feel guilt and shame, but rather humbly liberated and empowered from what I learned from my teacher's experience. I was infused with a dedicated focus to optimal health in every mental, physical, and spiritual facet. The profuse amounts of sweat dripping from my pores in hot yoga classes symbolized the release of negative feelings that I harbored within my body and mind. I was awakening powerfully to my true enlightenment. True enlightenment, I found, is the discovery of the unique powerful individual that you are and executing the desire that speaks to your true essence.

With the ancient practice of yoga that began in India over 5,000 years ago, I have absorbed it and applied it in accordance to my own Christian faith. It is the decision of the practitioner to decide what they may use the practice of yoga for. As an avid practitioner and teacher of yoga, it is my intention for all people everywhere to experience unprecedented levels of awakening and a place of wealth that includes joy, peace, and strength of mind, body, and spirit. The benefits of yoga are too great to explain; they need to be experienced. I encourage you in your quest for a successful body to give yoga a try and see what it can do for you.

About the Author

Sarah Jones' passion for yoga has allowed her to experience a free-flowing life of rhythmic expansion. She has now learned to possess daily gratitude, kindness, and forgiveness—attaining "yoga-licious" empowerment from within.

After the decision to obtain her 200-hour RYT and corporate chair yoga certifications, this led to the birth of Sarah's business, Fierce Bodhi LLC. With the combination of life lessons and the practice of yoga, she is now driven to lead others in corporate America through a vinyasa technique, so they too can experience a powerful awakening in their lives. She has a wide range of experience teaching people of all walks of life, locally and internationally.

Sarah's greatest strength is helping others reach the ultimate goal of discovering who they truly are as individuals and encouraging multitudes in raising the standards of the mind, body, and spirit.

Email: FierceBodhi@gmail.com
Website: www.fiercebodhiyoga.com

CHAPTER 13

CHRONIC INFLAMMATION: THE SILENT SABOTEUR

By Shira Litwack
Researcher, Chronic Care Manager, Medical Fitness Educator
Toronto, Canada

*The one unifying link between all diseases, mental and
physical is the presence of chronic inflammation.*
—Harvard Health

My goal in this chapter is to indelibly engrain chronic inflammation (CI) into
the number-one spot on your health watch. Instead of focusing on fitting into
our jeans, let's have fit genes.

According to the World Health Organization, chronic, noncommunica-
ble, and inflammation-related diseases are the largest cause of morbidity and
mortality globally.

Yet, sadly, chronic inflammation (CI) doesn't make it into the daily vernacular of health: we are changing that here. Chronic inflammation merits
the same fidelity as body fat, cholesterol, blood pressure. It is very real; it's not
kryptonite! By lowering our CI, we have a better chance staving off the pleth-
ora of mental and physical chronic inflammatory diseases that are out there.

More and more, researchers are challenging the paradigm that "growing
old" is a natural part of life. They believe it is a disease. From unravelling the
human genome, the conversation has evolved from "aging causes disease" to

"disease causes aging." As we will see, "aging" is not how many birthdays we've celebrated, it is how inflammation has conquered our cells.

Paving the Road to Hell with Good Intentions

"No way. He was such a health freak. How did this happen to him?" said all of us upon hearing the news of a "healthy" colleague who'd dropped dead.

We are constantly bombarded by "Eat this. Don't eat that. Exercise more. Take these vitamins. You should …" But, our orthorexic stringency could be paving the road by actually increasing chronic inflammation. On the surface, all looks great, but underneath we could be jeopardizing our health. As we get started on our quest to understand inflammation, I ask for open minds to challenge current quick-fix mantras and dig deeper into the root of what is happening in the human body to determine health and sickness.

What Is Inflammation?

Inflammation is our body's rescue response to perceived intruders such as infection or injury, a normal process to serve and protect. Damaged cells release chemicals triggering a response from the immune system. This is *acute inflammation*, a necessary immune response typically lasting hours to days.

Chronic inflammation (CI) happens when the normally protective role of inflammation becomes detrimental when the immune response becomes excessive in magnitude or duration. Two points to consider:

- Long-term inflammation can last for prolonged periods of several months to years.
- Because the stimulus of the immune system is continued, tissue destruction occurs, and function is diminished until lost.

Differentiating acute vs. chronic inflammation

Acute Inflammation	Chronic Inflammatory Diseases (CIDs)
Cuts	Autoimmune disease, asthma, COPD
Burns	Diabetes, macular degeneration, colitis, Crohn's
Frostbite	Cancers

Temporary infections

Allergic reactions

Bruised muscles

Broken bones

Heart disease

Depression and anxiety

Alzheimer's

Rheumatoid arthritis, sinusitis, periodontitis, neurodegenerative disorders, and BPH (prostate)

Information About Chronic Inflammatory Diseases

According to the National Institute of Health (NIH), worldwide, three out of five people die due to chronic inflammatory diseases (CIDs).

According to the NIH and the Center of Disease Control (CDC), the prevalence of diseases associated with chronic inflammation is anticipated to increase persistently for the next 30 years in the United States.

From "Chronic inflammation in the etiology of disease across the lifespan" December 2019: International experts from 22 research institutions including NIH, Stanford, Harvard, Columbia University Medical Center and University College London, agree inflammation-related diseases as the cause of 50 percent of all deaths worldwide. Conclusion: "Future research should focus on identifying ways to better diagnose and treat severe chronic inflammation."

Today, chronic inflammatory diseases are at the top of the list of death causes. There is enough evidence that the effects of chronic inflammation can be observed throughout life and increase the risk of death. It's no surprise that scientists' efforts are focused on finding strategies for early diagnosis, prevention, and treatment of chronic inflammation.
—Dr. Claudio Franceschi, world-renowned scientist, University of Bologna, Italy

Mental health is a vast concern. There is an abundance of research concluding that CI is equally at the root of these diseases.

Far from being specific to any one mental illness, or a subpopulation within a mental illness, inflammation turned out to be a common denominator and likely risk factor for every manner of psychiatric disturbance, from schizophrenia to obsessive compulsive disorder, from mania to depression.
—Dr. Miller, Medical Director *Psychiatric Times*

Covid-19 has changed our lives. I feel compelled to briefly share research: Why do some people recover, and others succumb? Research in this short time is telling us a cytokine (inflammatory agents) storm. According to the *Journal of the American Medical Association* (JAMA) Cardiology Studies in July 2020:

We've understood for a few months now that COVID-19 is not only a respiratory infection but a multi-system infection. There is an acute inflammatory response, increased blood clotting and cardiac involvement. And the cardiac involvement can either be due to direct involvement of the heart muscle by the infection and its inflammatory response …

Among 100 adults who recently recovered from COVID-19, 78% showed some type of cardiac involvement in MRI scans and 60% had ongoing inflammation in the heart …

The most common heart-related abnormality in the COVID-19 patients was myocardial inflammation or abnormal inflammation of the heart muscle, which can weaken it …

And yes … CI can lead to the demise of our furry friends as well.

Oxidative Stress to Chronic Inflammation

Oxidative stress (OS) is an imbalance between free radicals and antioxidants in the body, which leads to cell and tissue damage creating a state of chronic inflammation. Free radicals are oxygen-containing molecules with an uneven number of electrons (ROS). The uneven number allows them to easily react with other molecules. They can rob other cells of electrons, causing cellular damage, eventually leading to disease

Redox state is our balance between ROS (reactive oxygen species) and antioxidants. Note:

- We want to minimize our production of free radicals.
- We want to increase antioxidants to stabilize those free radicals, not just eating antioxidants we hear about, *but we want to increase our body's own ability to produce our own home-grown antioxidant system.*

Causes of Oxidative Stress and Chronic Inflammation: Endogenous vs. Exogenous

Endogenous sources (natural waste) of OS are normal by-products of cellular functions and production of ATP, a normal by-product of our metabolic activity.

Exogenous sources (external sources) of OS include smoke, alcohol, radiation, poor food choices, dehydration, over-exercise, lack of physical activity, adiposity, certain medications, chemicals, pollutants, rancid oils, stress, circadian rhythm dysregulation, infections, poor-functioning microbiome, and the list goes on.

It must furthermore be noted that CI diseases are on the rise. Why?

Our rapidly changing, demanding environment and choices we make increase oxidative stress. Our inner antioxidant defense system was not designed to manage the current burden. Our physiology is not optimized to our stress load.

The demand on our physiology from our very proinflammatory world and behaviors is far greater than our ability to combat this constant firing of inflammatory assaults. As an example, cell phones have become a necessity of our lives. I urge everyone to read up on the research on oxidative stress and cell phone usage. There are many studies ranging from "proceed with caution" to … much more dramatic conclusions that you should at least be aware of.

The Chicken or the Egg?

We are in a place where researchers can seriously ask the following questions: does aging cause disease? Or does disease cause aging? Which is it?

Aging ⇒ Disease   OR   Disease ⇒ Aging

This is truly the-chicken-or-the-egg issue of current research, but to many researchers of inflammation, aging is now called inflammaging!

The order of events seems to be: chronic exposure to OS ⇒ chronic inflammation ⇒ cellular malfunction, cell death, abnormal cell growth ⇒ aging.

Aging is a series of processes that include direct damage to cells and DNA and loss of information PLUS the accumulation of cellular waste, errors (epigenetics), imperfect cellular repairs, and the responses to those repairs.

Researchers on aging debate many theories and definitions of aging, all based on the demise of our cells. These various components of cellular damages are all collectively referred to as the "hallmarks of aging and disease". Researchers might disagree on the most influential cause of aging, but it is agreed, inflammation is the one constant, the trigger to cellular breakdown and dysfunction.

Epigenetics: AKA—Don't Blame Mama and Papa for Everything

Please forgive the brevity of this section; it really merits a full dissertation. However, a brief explanation is necessary to understanding how our choices and exposures create a proinflammatory state in the body.

Epigenetics: Tags on our DNA dramatically influence the way our DNA functions, for better or for worse. This is where lifestyle exposures affect our gene expression, our health. This explains why identical twins, born with the same genetic material, can age very differently, based on their environment and lifestyle choices.

First, there are epigenetic modifiers. These include:

- Diet—the way we choose to feed our body is a major epigenetic modifier, but interestingly, mom's diet during pregnancy is thought to cause epigenetic changes in offspring
- Obesity—fat cells release inflammatory cytokines
- Physical inactivity
- Smoking
- Alcohol
- Environmental pollutants
- Electric and magnetic fields
- Psychological stress
- Circadian rhythms

Epigenetics influences which genes are switched on (expressed), passing on the way the genes are used. In cancer, epigenetic tags can turn off tumor suppressor genes (TSG). The silencing of TSGs is an early driving force in the cancer process.

Soft inheritance: Epigenetic modifications remain as cells divide and can be inherited through the generations.

A point to ponder: what is the role of epigenetics in our evolution as a species?

Inflammation of the Gut

There is a strong relationship between gut health and overall health and vitality. Hippocrates said a mere 2500 years ago, "All diseases begin in the gut."

Inflammation in the gut leads to many of our chronic illnesses, mental and physical, plaguing our world. Every time we ingest anything—food, recreational choices—we should think about our mighty microbiome sometimes referred to as our "second brain."

Our microbiome, or our gut, can be a bacterial war zone between the good guys and the bad guys. Dysbiosis is a dysfunction in an imbalance of the gut microbial community by various stressors, pathogens, a sedentary lifestyle, etc. Dysbiosis promotes gut inflammation, and, if left unchecked, contributes to the development of chronic diseases such as inflammatory bowel disease (IBD), colon cancer, Alzheimer's, depression, obesity, neurodegeneration, asthma, autoimmune disorders, etc. Bad bacteria further upset our inner ecosystem releasing proinflammatory molecules.

Just how important is a balanced microbiome? Important enough to have fecal transplants (aka bacteriotherapy; aka poop in a pill!) Fecal transplants from individuals with a healthy flora are being performed to treat chronic intestinal infections.

The gut is truly Grand Central Station. Just to name a few things determined in the gut:

- Nutrient absorption
- Immune function
- Brain function
- Vitamin production
- Metabolic control
- Production of hormones including serotonin (our happy hormone)
- Hormonal control (yes, that fiery estrogen included)

The enteric nervous system (ENS) is the brain in our gut. It is known as the "second brain," and it can operate independently of the brain and spinal cord, our central nervous system (CNS).

One of the most fabulous people I have ever had the privilege of interviewing is Dr. Michael Gershon, the man who coined the term our "second brain." Dr. Gershon's 1998 book, *Our 2nd Brain, Our Belly Brain* is funny and brilliant. Amazing a book on the gut is so entertaining.

Researchers agree, gut health has a tremendous impact on our mental health and mood. Coincidentally, think about many expressions we use revolve around the gut:

- *My stomach is in knots*
- *Gutless*
- *Butterflies in my stomach*
- *Sick to my stomach*

We know the mighty microbiome is vital to immune function. Researchers look at how lowering gut inflammation can lower the risk of chronic inflammatory diseases (CIDs).

There are strong links between a loss of microbiota diversity as we age, as a potential contributor to chronic inflammation. Remember, "aging" is not necessarily how many birthdays were celebrated, but infers cellular breakdown, diseases, and disorders that lead to "aging." The gut microbiome is easily upset by inflammation, combined with declines in nutrient intake and absorption, contributing to a loss of healthy gut bacteria and function.

Leaky gut syndrome is an example. The gastrointestinal tract has four layers. The innermost layer is called the mucosa. The mucosa is both a physical and immunological barrier, keeping gut bacteria where they belong, preventing inflammation, and providing a controlled amount of inflammation in response to a pathogen or invader. Altered intestinal permeability causes leaky gut, opening the gates to inflammatory toxins to escape and circulate in the bloodstream. If you didn't guess, this is a bad thing.

How Can We Lower Our Levels of Chronic Inflammation?

From the NIH, we know that chronic inflammatory diseases account for more than 50 percent of deaths. Really, it is far more, but how can CI be controlled?

It can be controlled with how we feed ourselves and by our physical activity, the daily choices we make, and our awareness of our environmental stresses. Now let's rethink our health strategies from a proinflammatory perspective.

Food

It's not as you hope. No one can tell you, "Eat this, and you will lower your levels of inflammation." Sorry. According to Dr. David Sinclair, Harvard author of *Lifespan—Why We Age and Don't Have To,* "Science has demonstrated that the positive health effects attainable from an antioxidant rich diet are more likely caused by stimulating the body's natural defense against aging, including boosting the production of the body's enzymes that eliminate free radicals, NOT as a result of the antioxidant activity itself."

Food is an area where I urge people to not pave the road to hell with good intentions. Please be very careful consulting Dr. Google on "proinflammatory foods" and "anti-inflammatory diets."

There are a few dietary things we can do, however, to promote better health. First, the obvious. Limit or eliminate the following:

- Sugar and its various disguises, such as high fructose corn syrup and anything that breaks down into sugar
- Trans fats—studies show CRP (an accepted marker of inflammation) is dramatically higher in people who eat a lot of trans fats
- Excessive intake of omega 6 fats
- Refined carbs, high GI (glycemic index) foods, aka junk food
- Alcohol
- Processed foods—an often overused term—bacon, microwave popcorn, hot dogs, breakfast cereals, ready-to-eat meals, canned vegetables, etc.

I also encourage you to avoid very restrictive diets in the name of health, unless medically prescribed. I'm referring to diets that eliminate dairy, red meat, carbs. These are sources of precious nutrients that are bioavailable and are needed. Moderation, sources, and quality are all important factors in food choices. If we are going to eliminate a major food source, how do we receive those nutrients with the same bioavailability?

Red meat is a good example of how source and preparation are everything. Grass-fed vs. grain-fed, how it is prepared, frequency of consumption, fat, etc.—it isn't just about eating meat or not eating meat. It is the meat we eat that affects our health.

According to the NIH, with a study including 448,568 people, processed meat increased the risk of death while no effect was seen for unprocessed red meat. It is crucial to distinguish between processed and unprocessed meat, as the two can have vastly different effects.

Red meat and dairy can be full of hormones, antibiotics, and toxins depending on your country's laws. Unfortunately, certain countries also allow pesticides and genetic modification to crops. Be aware of sources.

Eating more fruits and vegetables, and plant-based diets are proven to lower CI, including promoting the body's own antioxidant defenses. However, this does not infer the total elimination of other potential nutrient sources.

According to the NIH, 2018: Both high and low percentages of carbohydrate diets were associated with increased mortality, with minimal risk observed at 50–55% carbohydrate intake

Alcohol

I am not the grinch, only the messenger.

There exist claims that a glass of wine a day is good for your heart. First of all, there are flaws in those studies. Secondly, can you think of other heart-healthy choices that don't use a known carcinogen and many other toxic chemicals? There are better ways to improve health.

The International Agency for Research on Cancer of the World Health Organization has classified alcohol as a group 1 carcinogen, similar to arsenic, benzene, and asbestos. The ethanol breaks down to acetaldehyde, which is a toxic chemical damaging DNA. It is abysmal how many everyday products contain alcohol.

Alcohol has ZERO nutritional value. It does NOT relax you; it fools you. Here are a few facts about alcohol:

- It is the lead suspect in gut inflammation.
- It disturbs the microbiota, increasing the permeability of the mucosa.
- It is an endocrine disruptor, toxins.
- It impairs multi-organ interaction.

- It leads to liver dysfunction.
- It can cause brain inflammation.
- It can lead to inappropriate behavior.

It is true that red wine has resveratrol, a potentially powerful antioxidant, not highly bioavailable, but drinking more wine won't help you become healthier. Let's do some simple math. To benefit from resveratrol, we need 40 mg to 500 mg per day. Red wine has 12.5mg per liter, so we need three to 40 liters a day to benefit from the resveratrol. No, this isn't the best solution.

Exercise

Exercise, by definition, is applying stress to the body. Exercise and physical activity are vital to our health, improving:

- Blood flow
- Lung and heart health
- Muscles (undoubtedly our BFFs in life)
- Telomeres
- NAD, a molecule vital for life

However, if you're just considering health, even exercise needs to be done in moderation. According to David C. Nieman in the *Journal of Sport and Health Science*, "High exercise training workloads, competition events, and the associated physiological, metabolic, and psychological stress are linked to immune dysfunction, inflammation, oxidative stress, and muscle damage." While, moderate and higher intensity exercise less than 60 minutes augmented immunosurveillance against pathogens and cancer cells and reduced systemic inflammation, which is good. After heavy exertion over 60 minutes (marathon), markers of adaptive and innate immunity were decreased, and markers of inflammation (cytokines) were dramatically increased. This is not good.

For optimal health, moderate exercise activities are encouraged. Embrace incorporating variety into your fitness routine so as to not always perform high intensity workouts. To help lower inflammation try: yoga, Tai Chi, meditation, range of motion, and Pilates are all good. And make deep breathing a regular part of your day!

Summarizing Choices and Exposures to Control Your Health

As knowledge of the causes of inflammation grows and the understanding that inflammation leads to certain avoidable diseases, anyone wanting a better health and a better body should be mindful of their choices from a perspective of CI. In this chapter, we've highlighted some—from smoking, to certain fats, to factors in our environment—but it isn't just things we have to go out and find that can harm us. Many everyday items like cosmetics, cleaning products, hand sanitizers, and lotions are absorbed through the skin and contain endocrine-disrupting chemicals that can lead to inflammation. Many countries have banned as many as 1,400 proinflammatory chemicals in cosmetics and personal care products, including those linked to cancer and reproductive and neurological disruption. As a planet, we have a long way to go, though. One score is about 1,300 to 11. That is 1,300 inflammatory products have been banned in Europe, and 11 have been banned in the US.

CI is like a venomous spider's nest spun from genetics, food, stress, activity, and environment. If we remain tangled in this web, our cells will break down, die, and fester. But unlike a fly in a web, we are not helpless victims to genetics. We can continue to fight diabetes, heart disease, depression, and cancer with medications, but we can also rip out the roots of CIDs. By lowering our levels of known saboteurs, we have a much better chance of staving off disease, having a happier, healthier life in tune with the successful body we live in.

About the Author

Shira Litwack is admittedly a science geek, who proudly hasn't read fiction since university. Shira has consulted in health for over 40 years, focusing on chronic care and recovery from disease by embracing the power of choice with nutrition, physical activity, and daily habits. Shira is privileged to have participated in numerous research projects on chronic inflammation and disease, sparking her to bring "oxidative stress" and "chronic inflammation" into daily vernacular with audiences.

Shira hosts a podcast, is interviewed by the media, and her raison d'être is educating people to measure and manage inflammation and feel the difference.

Shira has degrees in chemistry and psychology, over 20 fitness certifications, holistic nutrition, and addiction recovery. She has three grown successful sons, two beautiful dogs, and is blessed to still have her parents—the two best parents ever. She lives in the countryside on seven acres, where she works remotely with clients and audiences to uncover their fountain of youth.

Email: shira@BestInCorporateHealth.com
Website: www.BestInCorporateHealth.com

CHAPTER 14

SELF-TRANSFORMATION FROM THE INSIDE OUT

By Dee McKee
Mindfulness Business Coach, Transformation Coach
Melbourne, Australia

Create the highest grandest vision for your life
because you become what you believe.
—Oprah Winfrey

Would you like to have a toolbox that only you had the key to that would evolve your life into a peak state? One that would allow you to achieve your goals and dreams, and enable you to acquire the motivation to transform and have a better life? One that would allow you to obtain optimal health, physical fitness, and happiness with what you see in the mirror every day—your physical body? Would you like to create changes in your health and well-being while still having energy at the end of your day? Does this sound impossible? If so, then we are going to change this into a reality in this chapter. And, while we're at it, let's rewrite the next chapter in your life.

The secret to rewriting the next chapter of your life into the success story you desire is as simple as you believing everything that you need is already within yourself and everything on the outside is an illusion caused by your ego. Your body is your temple, you need to nurture it. You are the solution to manifest what you want. To produce the permanent changes that you truly desire, all you need to do is create the changes from within yourself.

Right now, what would the book of your life look like? How would the chapters read? Would they keep repeating themselves? Would all the chapters be the same? Are you going through the same motions every day, attracting the same outcomes? Are these outcomes what you want or not?

As we open the toolkit to lasting change, let's rewrite the chapters in your book. Let's learn about the empowerment that will allow you to shine and have the tools to create your own identity and create positive change in your life forever. Creating the change within yourself first will allow physical changes to follow.

One of the most important steps in creating lifelong changes is to learn to love yourself first and foremost. Loving who you are now and being comfortable in your own skin is key. You have one body and one life; it is your choice how you look after your body and how you choose to live in it. What choices are you currently making? Are you happy with these choices? How are your choices affecting not only you but the people around you? Knowing where you are is a big help in knowing what you want to change.

Gratitude

Creating change in your life can be helped by combining various elements into your day. Meditation, cardio training, strength training, yoga, Pilates, and good nutrition are among some of the activities we can embrace to generate positive changes. First, though, before embracing changes in those areas, the most important thing to embrace is gratitude: being grateful and being thankful for all we already have. Once we have gratitude for everything that we have in our lives right now, we begin to fight for ourselves, and this is the beginning of unlocking that toolbox. Begin to practise gratitude and thanks. Begin to look within yourself and you start to create new beginnings. Allow yourself to break through the chains and stop the negative cycle you are in, so you can change your unhelpful patterns into rewarding ones.

Showing gratitude because you think it is the right thing to do won't last, and you will fall back into old patterns. Rather, embrace the feeling of being grateful every day, and this feeling will radiate through your whole being. You can start by beginning each day with the simple task of writing three things that you are grateful for.

An example of someone who transformed through simple gratitude is one of my clients, Madison. Madison first came to me in a very dark place. Her life was not taking the direction that she wanted, and she was unhappy with how she was feeling and looking. After working with her, focusing on little things in her mindset, the changes were quite significant. In simply writing down what she was grateful for every morning, Madison came to realise all that she was truly thankful for in her life and how she already had so many wonderful things. Instead of focusing on what she did not have, she could now see all that she did have. This one change broke one of her harmful patterns and removed a block that she had held within herself for a long time.

Her positivity for her life started to change. Madison started to fuel her body in the correct way, and she hired a trainer and started to exercise. Her weight started to shift, and her body undertook a transformation. No longer did Madison feel the need to hide behind dark makeup and clothes; instead, she replaced them with light colours, which brought out the brilliance in her eyes.

People started to notice Madison's transformation and commented on how amazing she was and how they wanted to know her secret. The secret was simply that Madison was unlocking her toolkit. As she embraced her changes, she began to love herself more each day, and a newfound respect for herself formed. No longer was she unhappy. She had energy to complete the goals and plans she had set for herself.

Madison is now taking ownership of her destiny. She is creating her life and living her dreams. This change started with her removing just one emotional block. As we continued to work through her limiting beliefs, Madison grew stronger within herself. Nothing is stopping her from achieving what she wants in her life now, and she still starts each day the same way: meditation, being grateful, and setting her intentions for her day. These small actions create her success daily.

What if I told you that you create your mindset and even your feelings? That is what Madison did. Her example shows that what you think is what you become, so watch your thoughts. Thoughts control feelings and thoughts cause feelings. You are the creator of your thoughts and feelings. Let your thoughts drift a minute. Where do your thoughts drift to, and where do you feel they drift to? Now take the time and ask yourself the following: *what are my thoughts regarding my health? What are my thoughts around my appearance? How do I feel about the way I look? What am I saying to myself right now?*

Now, here is the important part to remember: what you say in answer to these questions is what you create. If you constantly think you will never look good, then you will never look good. If you say you will never lose weight, you are planting a negative emotion inside yourself and creating a block in your results. Remove the blocks from inside, and this will allow you to transform your body and become the best version of yourself, both physically and emotionally.

Meditation

Creating time in your day to relax allows you to visualise the beauty that is inside you. As mentioned earlier, everything that you need is already found within you to create the power of change. You can change your go-to patterns by changing your thought forms. You need to focus on what you can do and not on the can'ts. The second you focus on the "can't," your thought form changes and becomes a distraction, and within an instant you are back to thinking in your old patterns.

One of the easiest ways to change your thought form is through breathing. Meditation allows you to focus on your breathing, control your thoughts, and set your intentions regarding who you want to become or what you want to achieve. Meditation is a form of discipline that allows you to reprogram your patterns and work through your blocks. Whether you are a negative or positive thinker, remember, it is a choice. It is your choice.

The more quickly you can rejuvenate your thoughts and mind, the more quickly you will become whole. Calming your mind helps you calm your body and empower the creation of change. Meditation is a great way to start your day and can be done at any time throughout the day. This is an important tool that I have shared with many clients to enhance the qualities of their lives. Add gratitude into your meditation, and you start to create magic. Once we learn to be grateful for the little changes that we are achieving and love ourselves and our bodies for what and who we are, then the bigger changes begin to occur. It is now time to turn the key and unlock the power we have within and, above all, raise the expectations of our own self-worth.

Through the simple act of meditation and gratitude, you are releasing past life conditioning, and you begin moving from a lifeless state to your peak state. Moving forward and adding to the toolbox, you can add those various other elements around exercise and diet into your day. Before you add in these other elements, you need to remember the following lessons that will assist you in making the right choices for yourself: remember to be patient and kind to yourself; be aware of your old patterns; be ready for change; become the growth you deserve; and, most of all, be grateful for all that you learn on this journey. These tools will allow you to obtain the right combination so that you enjoy exercising and eating healthy, and these tools will allow the results to flow.

Meditation, as part of your daily routine, is about taking the time to honour yourself. Once this is a habit, you can add the exercise/fitness and nutritional elements to your day to continue working toward your successful body. These combined all impact your energy level and the physical results you will achieve. For your own well-being, you need to perform either cardio training, strength training, yoga, Pilates, or some exercise daily. This will aid in your total body transformation from the inside out.

Fuel

There is a saying, "You are what you eat," and there are no truer words said. To be able to perform at an optimal level both mentally and physically you need to provide your body with the right fuel source. Your body and your muscles are like a car engine. If you want premium performance, provide it with a superior product. If you want a second-rate performance, then provide it with a low-grade alternative. Your body is no different. For everlasting change and results, you need to change the way you look at your fuel intake. Providing your body with a quick snack on the run with no nutritional qualities is going to have you feeling tired and lethargic, and it won't provide you the power to last throughout the day.

Similar to fuelling a high-performance car with the best fuel, your body is also like a seed that you plant in the garden. You need to nurture it, provide it with sunshine, water, nutritional substance, and most of all, love, for it to sprout. Energy in and energy out is vital to the outcomes you want to achieve. To lose fat, you need to consume fewer calories than you expend, and to gain muscle you need to consume more calories that will help you to grow. Remember, though, you need to be fuelling your body with high-quality foods, foods in their natural forms are the best.

To become vigilant in treating your body like an expensive car or a cherished plant in your garden, prepare each meal. If your days are busy, plan a day when you can meal prep, so you can eat the foods that are best for your body rather than relying on the quick, less-nutritious options that are readily available. Meal prepping can be a key to the success of your body, and it can be part of something you can do with the whole family. Nutritional substance allows you to have the energy to complete the tasks in your day with effort and ease. It supplies you with mental and energetic stamina, giving you clarity instead of uncertainty.

What does your fuel cabinet currently look like? Is it due for an overhaul? Your muscles need the right fuel to thrive. Treat them with respect as part of your process in loving your body.

Movement

Your physical body honed through movement is the final part of your toolkit. The physical activities that you add to your day will greatly improve your overall well-being. These can be in many varied forms, and they must resonate with you to achieve the success you are after. It is important to add strength training exercise into your day to increase your muscle fitness. Fat is burnt up in your muscles, so the more muscle mass you gain, the more fat you will burn, not only through exercise but also during rest. Without strength training, you will lose muscle each year. This loss is a key factor in the decreasing of your metabolism. Only doing cardio-based exercises is not enough. For a maximised successful body, you need to incorporate the strength training element into your weekly routine, but it does not have to be difficult.

Adding body weight exercises, squats, pushups, lunges, and variations of these into your day is a great start. Weighted movements take time and should be performed at *your* level. Always reach out to a coach to assist you and set you on the right path. While gyms can be great, fitness does not have to be performed in a gym. You can exercise anywhere, at home, in the park, on the beach, wherever you are comfortable.

Yoga and Pilates are also fitness elements that can greatly enhance your transformation.

It is important not to judge yourself against anyone else when you are starting to exercise. Everyone is at a different point in their journey, and they are all following their own path. Judging yourself against others will allow negative self-chatter to come into your thoughts. Walking, running, cycling, swimming, skating—it all can be done to improve your fitness level. Finding something you enjoy is key here.

Remember when you were a child or when you watched a small child playing with boundless amounts of energy? Most likely, as a child, you would run and play for hours with no thoughts of being tired and with no thoughts of what other people were thinking about you. Why not play like a child again? You can be carefree and let your inner child come out and play each day. Jump in puddles, roll down that hill, do whatever your body is telling you it wants to do as long as you keep moving.

Learn to have fun within yourself. Be happy and become free. Free your mind from the negative and embrace the laughter. Make the change now as now is all that you have. Time is something you don't get back, so decide how you will use your time. Don't keep dreaming or blaming everything around you for you're not getting results. Look within yourself—that is where you start.

Take massive and immediate action in your life today. The choice is yours. Where are you going to place your focus today? Do you want to have a successful body?

Be grateful for all that you have, and the happiness you have inside will emerge. Happiness is the key to success, so step forward and radiate your powerful energy and feel peace rise within yourself, and your personal transformations will take shape from the inside out.

About the Author

Health, happiness, and success are important to Deidre McKee. Deidre, aka Dee, is a transformation coach, sales/business coach, and speaker who has spent over 30 years transforming people to be the best versions of themselves. Dee teaches that evolving your mind, body, spirit, and soul will allow you to transform yourself from the inside out. As a mum to her 7-year-old son, Jett, it is important for Dee to lead by example and make an impact on the world, one person at a time. Sharing love and gratitude and being continually thankful for everything are part of Dee's life, and she wants to share these things with you all.

Email: transformations@soul-ology.com.au
Website: www.soul-ology.com.au

CHAPTER 15
LINKING TO CREATE THE BEST AUTHENTIC YOU

By Shane McShea
Owner of The Fitness Society, Personal Trainer
Dublin, Ireland

I define success as being the best authentic me that I can be.
—Leeky Behrman, 9/11 survivor

A few years ago, I visited the World Trade Center in New York with my brother and dad. It was phenomenal. The building, the waterfall, the views over the city, the way the place was organised, the friendliness of the staff, and even the lifts were a spectacle—everything about the place is first-class.

Afterwards we went to a nearby bar for a drink, and Dad asked the barman a couple of questions—*how many visitors does the site get? How high is the building?*

The answers were between 15,000 and 30,000 visitors a day, and 1,776 feet tall. It was the 1,776 feet that really impressed us. Because those 1,776 feet are a deliberate representation of the year the United States Declaration of Independence was signed.

My brother and I are not usually stuck for words, but we found it hard to put them on the above figures and the monument itself. We thought of the huge amount of work which must have gone into everything to create and construct the World Trade Center (WTC) as it now stands.

A notable point that the barman made was how important it was to recover from the attack, honour its victims, and show strength despite the tragedy. This, the WTC definitely does.

So all the planning, the drawings, the cleaning of the site, the bricks laid, the steel put in place, the meetings, etc., were done with the overriding idea of both honouring the victims, and as the engineer of the project, Ken Gardner, said: "It stands for resolve, it stands for strength, it stands for renewal. To see the towers return would have an inspirational impact on the population".

At this stage, you may be wondering what this has to do with your health and fitness.

My answer—everything

As the project of rebuilding the WTC began, honouring the victims and providing inspiration moving forward must have been front and centre in the minds of all the people working on the project. This would have helped them push through the arduous meetings, criticism, stress, doubts, and sheer anxiety of the task in front of them.

So, all the gruelling planning, drawings, cleaning of the site, bricks laid, steel put in place can be linked to honouring the victims and providing inspiration moving forward. As a fitness professional, the parallels were immediately clear to me. Just like those rebuilding the Word Trade Center, to get the exact results you want, you need to be like the people working on the World Trade Center when it comes to your health and fitness—*know what you want to achieve and why you want to achieve it, and get genuinely excited about the journey you're on.* Then you can link all aspects of your fitness regime back to your "what" and your "why".

Let's talk about you. Maybe you are looking to lose weight, get stronger, improve your confidence. Maybe you are nervous about starting a gym program for the first time. Perhaps you are someone who is slightly sporadic about your health and fitness regime, and want to develop consistency. Or, you are someone who loves training and wants any further edge you can get. Regardless of your goal, my advice is to become absolutely clear on what's important to you and then link it to how being healthier and fitter can help you in that area. Below are some circumstances, including being a parent, a partner, and a professional, that show how examining how your fitness and health can affect others.

If you are a parent, surely, one of the very best things you can do for your kids is to inspire them around the benefits of being healthy and fit. Through your example, they will become as fit and healthy as they can by following your lead. On top of that, when you are at your peak, you will have more energy to spend quality time with your children. As a present, mentally alert, genuinely confident parent, you can lead them as well as being someone your kids and/ or nephews and nieces can be proud of.

Very often, parents will feel selfish if they spend time and money working on their health and fitness. In reality, spending this time and money is one of the least selfish things parents can do because it allows them so much more energy to be available to their family. A study by Duke Medicine published in the *International Journal of Obesity* in 2013 examined the relationship between the home environment and behaviours related to obesity. It found significant associations between a home environment and preschoolers' physical activity and their intake of healthy food versus junk food. The researchers concluded that to promote healthy behaviours in children, a healthy home environment and good parental role modelling are fundamentally important factors in generating healthy preschoolers. Maria Stroo, one of the researchers, stated, "It's hard for parents to change their behaviors, but not only is this important for you and your own health; it is also important for your children because you are a role model for them".

If you have a partner, whether that be a husband, wife, spouse, or significant other, it's a great feeling when you bring the best of yourself to the relationship. Your best might be being strong in the knowledge that you have taken control of something as important as your own health and mindset instead of letting circumstances or excuses control it for you. Also, if you're not in a relationship but would like to get one, coming from a place where you're feeling good in mind and body, and not looking for someone else to validate you, will work much better in the long run for all involved (written very much from experience!).

According to Aron, Norman, Aron, and Heyman in *Psychology Today*, lab studies in 2000 show that after jointly participating in an exciting physical challenge or activity, couples report feeling more satisfied with their relationships and more in love with their partner. I don't know about you, but with all of the pressures revolving around modern-day relationships, it seems like a bit of exercise to inspire this type of affection makes a lot of sense.

Now, if you're a professional working up the ladder of your career, then the energy, focus, resilience, and confidence built through an effective fitness routine is invaluable. If you're a manager, leader, or business owner, then that energy, focus, confidence, and resilience becomes even more important to drive your business forward and help inspire those working with you.

The following excerpt from Jim Kwik's book *Limitless*, which includes statements from Heidi Godman, executive editor of the Harvard Health Letter, shows how beneficial an exercise regime is to brain health: "Exercise changes the brain in ways that protect memory and thinking skills … Researchers found that regular aerobic exercise, the kind that gets your heart and your sweat glands pumping, appears to boost the size of the hippocampus, the brain area involved in verbal memory and learning."

Again, there is nothing complicated here. Just getting some exercise produces massive benefits, including benefits in the areas of memory and learning. This is another way to get ahead if you're interested in the success of your work or business.

Self-confidence is another area where exercise can create positive results. Self-confidence is a big one, and it is sad how many people have body confidence issues—regularly feeling uncomfortable in public settings as a result. A well-structured, consistent fitness regime will obviously be a big help in this area.

Most people have dealt with self-confidence at one level or another. Have you ever doubted yourself or been told you can't do certain things? Sometimes when I'm struggling with a workout, I will think of examples of when I've been told, "It's not happening," and I convince myself that if I can push through the session, it will help give me the mental and physical strength to prove wrong those who told me that, and sometimes that person is me.

Ultimately exercise has been shown again and again to help improve mood and confidence levels, and every successful workout you complete is a step towards you developing a mental image of someone who looks after your own health. You begin to appreciate your body, and when this happens, you are more likely to keep it up long term, continuing a positive physical and mental cycle in the process.

On top of all the benefits of exercise given above, what about your life span? How long do you want to live? If you ask me, life is kind of cool, and while none of us are guaranteed a certain amount of time here on Earth, a quick glance of the internet will give you an insight as to how useful exercise is as an anti-ageing agent. Amongst the potential benefits, you'll see how exercise can help boost your immune system, help prevent the development of certain cancers, strengthen bones to lower the risk of osteoporosis, and help protect your cardiovascular health. So, another great result of some often-enjoyable movement of your body is to help you stick around longer. That has to be considered a pretty good cost-to-benefit.

Linking—Use It for Anything

As I write about being a parent, a partner, a professional, and about having self-confidence and living longer, there is something that ties all of this together, and it is *linking*. In essence, the concept of linking can be used for anything. Linking involves tying things together in a way that will help you, that will motivate you. You may say, "It's easy for a personal trainer and gym owner to talk about connecting when it comes to health and fitness", but the reason I'm so passionate about linking is because I use it all the time for myself. Here, let me explain more about linking.

My first time really hearing about linking in a structured manner was at a John Demartini presentation where he taught the benefits of linking things you don't like doing to things you do like. In the years since, I've used linking to work harder in jobs, to help more people get results, to own my own fitness facility where people can get fitter, healthier, and happier in a fun, effective environment.

Linking has given all of the following a new meaning to me: every 5 am start, every cleaning of every toilet in the gym, every late-night work time, all the stress, and every one of the books I read. Linking has made them much more enjoyable as a result. Since I discovered linking, even reviewing accounts is something I look forward to now, and this is something I hated in the past. Now I see linking as a necessary step towards anything I want to achieve.

Obviously looking after my health and fitness is going to be a huge part of the journey because it's something I love to do, but anytime I don't feel motivated to train, by using linking, I can connect my workout to something bigger in my life that's more important than the workout but that doing the workout will certainly influence for the better. For example, I can link the workout to being a better uncle, to being a more confident business owner, and to bringing positive energy into my relationship. With linking, I literally think about how the one workout in front of me will improve the quality of my life, and I keep this up from workout to workout. Linking allows us to connect seemingly discreet acts to our big-picture goals, which, in turn, provides motivation.

For you to put linking to use, the best way is to take some time to figure out what is really important to you in life and figure out how being at your best fitness-level and best mindset will help you grow in the area. Once you decide this, create an effective health regime for yourself, and get help putting one together for your goals if necessary. Then it's a case of building the quality habits into your daily routine and all the while keeping yourself aware of the links between being fit and healthy to the areas in your life you want to progress in.

Once you see how your life will improve with better fitness, then all of the planning you put in, every rep you complete, every vegetable or glass of water you consume, every walk or run you go on, the mindset work you do, all of the unhealthy temptations you avoid, and the healthy habits you gravitate towards will come together for you as important steps in your own personal project. You'll be developing the plans, laying the foundations, putting the bricks in place, developing your own resolve, your own strength, and your own renewal. Ultimately, you'll be giving yourself the best thing that anyone can have—*creating the best authentic you that you can be.*

About the Author

Shane McShea is a Personal Trainer and owner of The Fitness Society gym in Dublin, Ireland. He strongly believes that people should be made aware of the multitude of benefits of a healthy lifestyle and be encouraged to lead a life that they enjoy. The Fitness Society's vision is to help everyone who comes to work out with them to get fitter, stronger, and healthier in a fun, effective environment.

Email: info@thefitnesssocietyireland.com
Website: www.thefitnesssocietyireland.com

CHAPTER 16
MOTION IS LOTION

By Jenna Minecci
Injury and Rehabilitation Specialist, Personal Trainer
Atlanta, Georgia

*Excellence is an art won by training and habituation. We do
not act rightly because we have virtue or excellence, but we
rather have those because we have acted rightly. We are what we
repeatedly do. Excellence, then, is not an act but a habit.*
—Aristotle

"Motion is lotion!"

I heard this for the very first time in college from my mentor Jenny
Moshak, former head athletic trainer for the University of Tennessee Lady
Volunteers. Looking back, it seemed like this was just a silly catchphrase. I
didn't realize the impact and power it would have over my life and over my
influence on others' lives. As I dove deeper into my kinesiology major in college, I realized this catchy phrase was true mentally, physically, scientifically,
and emotionally. It was the core and essence of being a human. It encompassed
the truest path to health, happiness, and longevity.

At the time, having endured six major knee surgeries, I wasn't totally
convinced moving more could truly help me. Moving hurts! How could this
be beneficial?

Pain triggered me to be anxious and upset. It seemed that my physical pain
created even more mental anguish. It fostered feelings of doubt and insecurity

about myself and my abilities. I was a devout soccer player as a kid and ended up tearing my ACL on both of my knees during my freshman and sophomore years of high school. After having surgery, and entering into a grueling reha-bilitation process, I learned shortly after my second surgery the harsh reality that both of my surgeries were performed improperly, and I required two more. It was devastating, and unfortunately, it led to six surgeries by the time I was in college, and nine surgeries by the time I was 30 years old. My fascination with fixing my own pain and preventing further surgeries helped me to realize "motion is lotion" for both the mind and the body. Living in pain physically leads to living in pain mentally, and the only way to turn this vicious cycle around is to control your mindset and move more.

Motion is lotion. Think about it. Humans are the most biomechanically fascinating creatures. Movement is at the core of everything in our lives, from the most exciting forms of entertainment to the core of activities where we find joy and peace. It is no coincidence that humans evolved based on our ability to move. Foraging for food and tracking our prey was only the beginning. Once we learned how to run and cover large distances of the world around us, we began to migrate, settle the entire planet, and likewise we became smarter. Humans have a muscular and skeletal system that allows us to move in more diverse and complicated patterns and sequences than any other living thing. With complex movements, the brain has to comprehend different sequencing and, in turn, master new tasks, ways to hunt, and live.

Exercise, movement, or just getting the heart rate up in general primes brain cells with oxygen. This act of work-enabling oxygen actually catalyzes the growth of new brain cells as well as the production of factors that aid in the creation of new synapses. These new synapses help the body to remember the new thing that was learned. The more complexly we began to move, the smarter we became. See where am I going here? From the perspective of phys-ical advancement, the brain is movement. Humans have the ability to move in more ways than any other animal, and we are the smartest of all animals; this is no coincidence.

Yet, as we come up with more technology, we begin to become more sed-entary than ever before. There are extreme obesity issues in many countries around the world, and the injury risk for younger athletes continues to increase as they adapt to a more habitual sedentary lifestyle. We also are living in more chronic pain than ever before because we aren't moving enough.

So how does this play into our actual joints and help with pain? Most of the large joints in the human body are synovial joints. Synovial joints are special because a natural lubricant is excreted into that joint called synovial fluid, which helps to cushion and aid the joint. But the catch is, this synovial fluid is only excreted with, you guessed it, movement. Not only does moving more help your brain to fire at optimum efficiency, but it also assists in a natural pain management system for our joints; hence, motion is lotion!

Now we need to put movement and brain power together in order to improve our mental health. It can feel impossible when everything hurts, you are feeling depressed, and the last thing you want to do is go exercise, but it truly can be the best thing for you. Daily exercise and even diverse movements can help tremendously with your well-being and mental health. Walking, dancing, hiking, canoeing, yoga—the list goes on and on. Any doctor will tell you that movement is essential to fight stress and stay positive, but how do you do all this when it hurts to move, and you are scared?

When I was a teenager, I hit an extremely low point in my surgery journey. Everything hurt, I never had any fun because I was stuck lying in bed recovering from surgeries all the time, and I missed my old, normal life. You know, the life where I was able to move and not rely on my mother to bring me food, help me take a shower, or use the restroom. No one could help me; heck, no one I knew could even relate to me. After throwing myself a major pity party, getting extremely angry and jealous while trying to watch the World Cup, and ultimately feeling like I wanted to give up, I finally realized it was on me. I had to overcome it. I had to solve it, so I could be me again, and that required figuring out how to move enough to do my rehabilitation. Those were the only things in my control.

I began silently reciting "Patience, persistence. Patience, persistence, Patience, persistence," over and over again in my head. I heard it in a rap song on the radio and recalling it made me feel a little emotional. Those lyrics were the first feeling of positive hopeful emotion I had felt for a long time. At first, it felt awkward, but soon I started to feel a little emotion again, a little ambition, a little tingle inside of my soul. I started whispering, "Patience, persistence." It felt good. I could feel a little twist in my heart, a small change of emotion causing me to feel joy and fear all at once. To my surprise, there was still something in there. I kept going. My whisper turned into a louder and louder chant until finally I was screaming it at the top of my lungs: "PATIENCE, PERSISTENCE! PATIENCE, PERSISTENCE!" I began to smile and feel like myself again. I continued to repeat this phrase as I completed my rehabilitation for the day, and I realized a few things: I felt better, I didn't hurt as much, and I took control over my thoughts to create positive change. Even if it was small, it was there, and I had unlocked the secret.

A few years later, when I heard Jenny Moshak coach her trainers and athletes on the philosophy "motion is lotion," it just clicked. I had empowered myself to keep moving, and sometimes that's all you can do. It was a huge victory, and it will be an ongoing part of life—facing setbacks and continuing to move forward. I knew the little phrase, "Motion is lotion," would change my life, just as "Patience, persistence" had in my darkest moments.

As a young adult, I faced an even more difficult surgery journey including bone grafts and multiple back-to-back surgeries. This was a challenging time in my life because not only was I faced with these immense physical and mental challenges again, I was almost bankrupt from surgeries, and I was living alone, without my mother to assist me and without any certainty that these surgeries would even help me. At that same time, my friends were going through master's degree programs, getting married, and having babies. It felt like everyone was doing something really special and incredible with their lives, and here I was, still having surgery, still stuck in the same place I was fifteen years before.

I immediately turned to the blame game and the feeling of helplessness: "Why me? What did I do to deserve this? Where is my joy and happiness?" And this time, "Patience, persistence" wasn't enough. This time, I knew I needed to truly use all my knowledge and experience from my career and from my previous surgeries to pull myself through this. I understand my immediate reaction of pity and shame was natural, given the situation, but it was also 100 percent in my control. If I had learned one thing from my previous surgeries, it was that I control my own thoughts, feelings, and reactions. I had to change how I perceived this challenge, or it would break me; and I had come too far, fought through too many surgeries, to give up here.

I began to prepare, knowing my mindset was going to be just as important as my movement. As I had learned previously, my body fueled my mind and my mind propelled my body. I developed a program involving small amounts of safe movements that coincided with mindset work, specifically positive affirmations. Initially after surgery, this was only small amounts of movement, like taking a slow and safe stroll around my apartment on my crutches or moving my arms around in different, fun patterns just to get my heart rate up and my blood pumping while my legs and body were resting. It might sound silly, but this was actually pretty fun considering I couldn't do much else after having major surgery. I realized my perspective changed from "I can't do anything" to simply appreciating the little movements I could do and focusing my energy on gratefulness. Every hour or two while I was awake, I would do some of these simple things, and over time, it became filled more and more with stretches and other safe rehabilitation techniques I was able to add as I progressed. I fed my body with movement, and it instantly rewarded my mindset with hope and focus.

I used this new perspective to develop a mental routine too. Every morning, as soon as I woke up, I would write down a list of positive affirmations. At the beginning, I wasn't very good at being vulnerable (even with myself), and my affirmations weren't the best, but over time I realized how effective they were and the affirmations evolved into long lists. The fun part is, you can create your own affirmations, and they can be about anything: life, relationships, breaking habits, loss. All you need to do is start with "I CAN," "I AM," and "I WILL." Try to design statements that are specific to what you are going through this year or even just today. Here are some examples. *I am strong and ready to grow. I can take things one day at a time. I will ace my interview and find my dream job. I am beautiful, confident, and feminine. I can be anything I want to be. I will conquer surgery and come out stronger and smarter. I am in control of my own self-worth. I will choose greatness today. I am grateful for my body. I am beautifully and wonderfully made. I am calm and at peace. I will play soccer again. I am stronger than my fears.*

When I returned back to work, I started carrying around my daily list of affirmations because different challenges and difficulties regarding my injuries would make me upset. If I had a negative emotion, I would quickly walk outside or excuse myself to the restroom and pull out my affirmations. By realizing when I was creating negative energy and immediately changing my thoughts, I truly changed my life. My affirmations were ready for me at any moment, even a moment of weakness and negativity. We all have moments or days like this, no one is perfect. But it takes consistent effort to constantly be in control of our thoughts in order to continue to create positive energy.

It's now been three years since I began my mindfulness journey. These techniques that I adapted through necessity during surgeries have helped me in a multitude of situations in my life. "Motion is lotion" fuels my body, my workouts, my rehabilitation, and my perspective. I spent one full year writing daily positive affirmations and prioritizing daily movement, and I still can't believe the greatness I achieved with such simple methods. I pledged to myself to continue this forever. I am grateful for my body and my journey because without either, I would have never truly learned the real purpose for my body and mind.

No matter how bad things are in our life, or in the world as a whole, let's remember that everyone experiences difficult, or seemingly unbearable, situations. Let's also remember that as long as we manage to keep our minds and bodies moving forward during exasperating times, and we apply positive affirmations to help us stay focused on what we can control, then that is where our true happiness lies.

Never give up. Never stop moving. Motion is lotion.

About the Author

Jenna Minecci is a passionate personal trainer and strength coach dedicated to helping others prevent injury, prepare for surgery, and recover exceptionally from any surgery they have. After having four ACL reconstructions fail on her as a teenager, she has now had nine surgeries and counting. Her goal is to educate and empower others facing difficult surgeries and recovery journeys. She specializes in corrective exercise, knee rehabilitation, and ACL injury prevention. Jenna is also the author of the book *Surviving 7: The Expert's Guide to ACL Surgery* available on Amazon. Follow Jenna on social media, @Jennactive, or email to learn more about her offerings, jminecci@gmail.com.

CHAPTER 17

YOUR BODY IS YOUR AUTOBIOGRAPHY: EMOTIONS, PERCEPTIONS, BELIEFS, AND WELL-BEING

By Selena Ella Moon
Psychosomatic Practitioner, NLP Master, Reiki
British Columbia, Canada

You have the power to heal your life, and you need to know that.
—Louise Hay

Hello there, it's a pleasure to meet you in the pages of this book. It is no accident you're reading this right now, and I hope to offer you a new perspective of your health that, perhaps, you have never before considered.

The perspective I offer is derived from my studies in biology, psychology, psychosomatic therapy, neuro linguistic programming (NLP), and energy healing. On top of that, I have two years of experience as a personal trainer certified in TRX, CrossFit, exercise and program design, and fascial stretch therapy. I also took it upon myself to get certification in a dietary program, originating from Germany, called Metabolic Balance.

Throughout the past decade in the time I've spent working with clients to improve their lives and overall health, I noticed some interesting discrepancies between what is shared in mainstream media about health and my client case studies, and this is something I'll go into more in this chapter.

What Contributes to Good Health?

To many people, their state of health is simply a direct reflection of what they eat and how much they move. This is something we have been taught to for quite some time. The Western world has put an emphasis on diet, supplements, and exercise programs to help people feel better, look better, and experience better health.

Based on my own experience, and client explorations, I believe the Western notion of health holds true to a significant degree, but I have also found that a person's emotional state, experiences, belief systems, and closest relationships also significantly impact their health. Doctors may classify these factors as "stress." However, after diving into the aspects of how stress is manifested through the chakra system in the human body, I want to ensure you understand that the human experience caused by the factors around us is much more complicated than blanketing emotional states with the primitive term "stress."

We, as humans, carry within us an array of solidified beliefs about food, movement, our bodies, the environment, and the earth. These beliefs often take hold by the time we are 7 years old. Much of the way we interact with our bodies and our eating patterns emerge from the continuous witnessing and modelling of those who immediately raised us. For example, if we watched Mom or Dad eat sugary foods when they felt pressed for time, then we may be apt to behave in the same way.

In addition to being molded by our child-rearers, we also form beliefs about our bodies based on how the outside world interacts with us. As children, we can be quite sensitive to the opinions and judgments of others, and often internalize criticism and belief systems that others' around us hold. If you have a friend or family member, whose opinion you value, speak unkindly about your body, you may form a rejection of your own self over time. This can lead to major issues relating to self, which can subsequently cause you to turn towards extreme behaviors that are unhealthy and emotionally damaging.

In my time as a personal trainer, I had the opportunity to consistently run blood tests on my clients through the Metabolic Balance Nutrition program for which I was simultaneously coaching. I realized that many of my "skinny" clients came out with more imbalances in their blood work than did my "overweight" clients. These results led me to believe that our health is about much more than what we weigh. This was contrary to what I had been taught, and it opened my curiosity so much that I entered the world of psychosomatic therapy, the study of how our emotional experiences and perceptions directly impact our physical body.

The Role of Experience, Emotions, and Perceptions on Our Health

After completing my level 2 psychosomatic practitioner program from the Australasian Institute of Psychosomatic Therapy, I was floored by how much of what I learned was directly applicable to the lives of my clients' and to my own life when it came to understanding the body.

I will now share some fascinating examples with the intent of opening your mind to the possibility that there is much more at play beyond diet and exercise when it comes to our overall well-being and physical symmetry.

Case Study 1—Heart Chakra

When I worked as a personal trainer, I had a male client who was having difficulty putting muscle on his chest. His back, arms, and shoulders were gaining muscle rapidly; however, no matter how good the exercise program was for building muscle, the client struggled with keeping it on his body.

After coming back from my psychosomatic therapy course, I learned that the chest area is associated with the heart chakra. This chakra is connected to love, compassion, forgiveness, grief, and giving and receiving. This led me to ask some more personalized questions to him, and to no surprise, I discovered this client had lost his father early in life and had never quite healed from the grief. This was causing a constriction of energy in his heart and blocking him from adding muscle to his body in that region. I decided to attempt some neurolinguistic programming tactics with him. After initiating a trigger release at the point of his diaphragm, we were able to get the energy flowing back into his heart.

Typically, when a major blockage is released from the body, a person's deeply numbed emotions will surface, and a lot of crying and purging must take place before moving forward in life with better alignment. This process was initiated with this client, and he took some time away from the gym to let himself feel and heal. When he returned to the gym, I was no longer a personal trainer, but I was aware of positive results regarding his ability to build muscle in his chest.

Case Study 2—Sacral Chakra

After becoming certified as an energy healer and emotional release trigger point therapist, I worked with a variety of clients who were interested in healing beyond losing weight or gaining muscle. This led me to a particular client who was having difficulty getting pregnant.

Fertility is connected with the sacral chakra, and this had me exploring her body for any pain, numbness, or energy blockages that were apparent. Again, to no surprise, I discovered a region in her lower back, which is where the sacrum is located, that was harboring intense beliefs around the concept of a child being a burden. I was able to use my clairvoyant and clairaudient gifts to communicate directly with the cells in her body that were carrying these inherited beliefs from her mother and clear them both through trigger release as well as energy work. Within two weeks of our session together, the client became pregnant.

Case Study 3—Kidney Stone Love Letter

Over the past four years, having the ability to shift energy at a distance, I have spent the majority of my time working with clients online. I was recently introduced to a client who had been diagnosed with kidney stones, and she did not want to surgically have them removed.

After entering her energy field, I was able to see that there were a few things happening emotionally and perceptually that were not allowing her to naturally pass the stones. The first was a feeling of anger towards her own feminine reproductive system, and the second was a total dissociation from the sacral region of her body. In order to heal, we must first find appreciation and love for our body, as it is perfectly designed with its own intelligence to help us heal and restore balance organically.

While speaking with her, I discovered she was told from a young age that if she wanted to have children, her child would be deformed due to the epilepsy medication she was prescribed to stop her from having seizures. Since she had not been taught how to process her emotions in a healthy way, the emotional impact caused her body to take on the burden resulting in the development of kidney stones.

Only two days after her first session, she lost five pounds and the symptoms of her stones were beginning to go away. In continuing to work with her, I had her write a letter to her kidney stones with love, acknowledging their presence in her body and letting them know she is processing the emotions of not being able to conceive. This gave the kidney stones permission to begin leaving her body without force and rejection, but with grace and appreciation. It is important to remember that our body is living, alive, and very susceptible to the information we give it with our thoughts. Much more than most people think, our mind communicates with our body with either harmful or positive messages, and with either, our body will react.

Every cell in our body stores consciousness, and our body reflects back to us the things we are telling it. If we tell our body, "You are bad, and you keep making me suffer," the body will take this as a command to continue pain. However, if we tell our body, "I acknowledge your genius and know you are serving a purpose that I am open to learning," we create an opening, a dialogue to learn more about the way our body is operating and why. In doing this, we release the resistance and flow of life happening through us, and allow for transformation and healing to occur.

Case Study 4—Sciatica and Vulnerability

I remember moving to a new city, a new home, and starting a new life after hosting over 200 events and workshops in a span of three years. I needed to take a break, and I was burnt out. I grew so accustomed to being a "teacher" and using my gifts and knowledge to help others, I had totally dissociated from what it meant to be a vulnerable and flawed human, myself. Soon after my move, I began experiencing shooting pain down my legs and the side of my back. I went to the doctor to discover I had manifested sciatica.

Upon doing some research, I realized that sciatica is connected directly to being extremely prideful and not asking for help. At the time, this was exactly the type of person I had become. So much of my ego needed validation from helping others, I could hardly work up the courage to ask for help when I needed it.

I began combining a program that a physiotherapist had offered me alongside a series of applicable affirmations I would recite every morning. Some of these affirmations included: *I allow myself to receive love and support. I am deserving of receiving help from others. Asking for help makes me more powerful, not less. When others offer support, I say yes. I allow myself to speak honestly and share my vulnerability with people I trust. I invite a network of people whom I can rely on.* I also became mindful of when I was acting prideful and began to change my behavior patterns to become a more vulnerable and authentic receiver of the support I desperately needed at the time.

Within 60 days, my sciatica was completely gone and has not returned since.

Patterns of Health as They Relate to Experience and Emotions

Prior to leaving you and concluding this chapter, I'd like to share some overall themes and patterns I have seen in clients to help you identify potential root causes of health challenges you may be facing. Albeit brief, this list may assist you in coming to terms with your emotions and how they may be impacting your health. If nothing else, my goal in showing you this list is for you to, at least, consider how perception and emotional factors might be manifesting in your body in various ways.

- Difficulty dropping fat—emotional suppression
- Prostate cancer—feeling sexual shame
- Hashimoto's disease—inability to speak up properly for yourself
- Lower back pain—feeling a lack of security in a relationship or financially
- Kyphosis—hurt from a past relationship and trying to protect your heart
- Acne—disliking oneself
- Bloating and gas—undigested ideas
- Diabetes—feeling a lack of sweetness in life
- Deafness—not wanting to hear
- Eyesight—not wanting to see things clearly
- Parasites—letting others live off your energy

If you would like to learn more about the correlations between physical ailments and emotional root causes, I highly recommend Louise Hay's book *You Can Heal Your Life*. The book offers a very comprehensive introduction to what I am referring to here as psychosomatic therapy and has helped millions of people connect more deeply with their true self and heal.

Concluding Statements

I hope this chapter has inspired you to explore your body and your health in a way that allows you to engage with your emotions, beliefs, and perceptions about life. I find this work extremely empowering, as it puts the control back in your hands. It is possible for you to shift your ideologies and reprogram your subconscious mind for success and happiness in the long term. Although this is not a replacement for Western medicine, psychosomatic therapy is most certainly potent information that can be used to help us harmonize our bodies and live longer, more fulfilling lives.

I have had the pleasure of speaking at conferences for functional medicine doctors, chiropractors, and other health practitioners who have opened their minds to the possibility that there is much more to life than what we can physically see. I personally began this journey with a scientific degree in biology and have been able to exponentially increase my capacity to serve humanity by combining my scientific knowledge with emotional awareness and the utilization of spiritual gifts.

If you are struggling with a particular health concern and are having difficulty pinpointing and healing the root cause, please don't ignore it. Reach out and get help. You can get support through your healing journey. I want to remind you that it is safe for you to explore your emotions and to face them head-on, despite whatever society has demonstrated or taught you. I promise you: you will find great power by allowing yourself to face your pain and move through it.

Each and every human being experiences emotion, and there are plenty of tools available now to find safety in this exploration. If we remain disconnected from the way we feel, we will never truly find happiness, and happiness is what breeds health in the body. My advice is to start small, and in each moment, practice asking yourself, "How does this make me feel?" In doing so, you will begin connecting more with your emotional body, and over time, you will have a grander perspective of what is taking place deep within.

Thank you for reading. I wish you infinite health and youthful living as you expand past your current limitations and enter into your perfect body.

About the Author

Selena Moon has been supporting clients in personal transformations for over a decade. As a psychosomatic therapist, master NLP practitioner, and energy healer, Selena has helped hundreds of clients internationally to identify the root causes of their personal challenges and create positive changes in their health, relationships, and careers. Selena has facilitated hundreds of workshops, events, and retreats, offering her participants insights, healing tools, and immediate opportunities to shift out of old thinking paradigms blocking health, happiness, and success.

Selena's greatest strength is her intuition, which she uses to identify and assess individuals on a personal level. Her private online sessions are uniquely tailored based on the client's individual circumstance. Selena uses a holistic approach, combining spiritual practices with scientific awareness and subconscious programming to initiate positive changes. Selena often also uses visualization techniques in her workshops and sessions, and she can help you. Contact Selena directly to receive a complimentary 20-minute consultation from Selena herself.

Email: theselenamoonproject@gmail.com
Website: www.selenaellamoon.com

CHAPTER 18

THE INNER JOURNEY FROM SHAME TO SUCCESS

By Kealah Parkinson
Communications Coach, Host of Tune In:
Radio for Your Mind, Body & Soul
Chicago, Illinois

The Universe is not outside of you. Look inside yourself;
everything that you want, you already are.
—Rumi

Mindset is everything.

Is it really? What do you think?

Do you dismiss that as a flat platitude? Do you check your mental box, "I already know that," and move on? Or do you start to mentally punish yourself with thoughts like, "Gosh, I'm so stupid! I *know* this, but I keep forgetting to practice it"? If you answered yes to any of these, you may want to rethink what you *think* you know about mindset.

Healthy skepticism, something that can be a valid piece of any of these example responses, carries some form of curiosity, as opposed to outright rejection, which is now known, thanks to psychologist Carol Dweck, as "fixed mindset." But the title "fixed mindset" is a little misleading: this "fixed" belief system, like all beliefs, is actually something that can be changed.

Take James as an example. As a child, his mother often introduced him to new people by saying, "This is James. He's shy. Say hello, James." With the label "shy" fixed firmly in place, you can probably guess what came next.

James would often hide behind his mother or involuntarily turn his face away from the people he was being introduced to, look at the ground, and mutter a greeting. James's developing brain did not learn social skills or any sense of overcoming the shy feeling that typically overcame him in new situations. Instead, it *fixed* on the idea, "I am shy." As an adult, James struggled to fit into his job description when his role suddenly extended to include some outside sales. Motivated by money, he voraciously read Zig Ziglar, Dale Carnegie, and Napoleon Hill. At this, James was inwardly thrilled to learn that he could overcome the belief that he was permanently, cripplingly shy. With these tutors in his briefcase, he practiced eye contact, firm handshakes, genuine smiles, and repeating and remembering his prospects' names. At home and around his neighborhood, he was still that shoe-gazing mumbler he'd been as a child, but at work, James was a standout salesman with top performances. What was the difference?

In another case, Emily was a child who also displayed shyness. Emily's mommy was a proponent of neuroplasticity. Emily's mom didn't study online or read books about childhood neurodevelopment. She simply knew that she, herself, had been shy as a child but had overcome it when given opportunities to practice social skills, even with making little blunders without ridicule. As a mother, she simply gave her child the chance to do likewise.

"This is Emily," she said to new people. When the little girl inevitably hid, looked away, or muttered, her mother would smile and let her—and sometimes gently ease her into new territory. Once, for example, she bent down to Emily and said kindly, "I'm not sure they can hear you when you speak so softly. Can you speak up a little?" Her daughter raised her voice and automatically lifted her posture.

To make her feel even safer, her mother frequently chatted with Emily on the ride home: "You felt a little shy when you met your new friend today, didn't you? It's okay to feel shy. You always get over it and feel better when you get to know them, don't you?"

Emily's self-concept was adaptable. The guidance she received from her mother encouraged it. James's self-image was also adaptable, but early on, he had no obvious guiding support system to let him know this.

Until recently, the overall wisdom on intelligence was that people were born with an IQ, or intelligence quotient, and that it more or less remained fixed throughout their lifetimes. Emerging data in the last couple of decades has debunked this. Many schools and workplaces have come to view the human brain as able to learn through every age and stage of life. Instead of viewing people as stuck at one level of IQ (fixed), the more progressive groups tend to look at the environment surrounding individuals to see if small changes can help bloom adaptability. After all, organizations can be fixed or growth-oriented too, with the leaders representing the "brains" of the body, or team members.

Let's look again at James and Emily. James came from a community with rigid rules and high expectations, many of them culturally imposed as traditions. His parents didn't love every aspect of this, but they had never known otherwise or even that the option to do differently existed. They passed on to their son, well-meaningly, what they had been taught: *some people are shy. Some are outgoing. Some members of the community are smart. Some not. Everyone has a talent, but some talents are valued more and help more people. Some people, like James and his parents, are meant to serve in silence in small spaces*, it seemed.

When James seemed to break the mold in adulthood, no one in his home or family was actually aware of it. They knew he had gotten a promotion and a raise but had no idea he'd broadened his skill set leading to that outcome. At home, he continued to fit their socially shy expectations. His view of himself, in fact, remained unchanged. James still considered himself shy but thought he had mastered a business skill, one that apparently didn't translate to backyard barbecues.

By contrast, Emily started to seek out opportunities to practice her new skills, first in her classroom, then in extracurricular activities as an adolescent. Because no one was coercing her into these steps, she took full responsibility and believed in herself to a greater degree than others.

Emily used a type of self-propelled growth mindset that later evolved into "positive disintegration"—that point in an individual's human evolution where she identifies personal liabilities, then moves away from the basic needs of sleep/food/shelter and social acceptance toward a more individuated, individualistic motivation: the need for self-actualization to become the best version of yourself.

Emily's results were such that, at one point, in her late 20s, while working a high-profile, well-compensated position at a globally known non-profit organization, she encountered what felt to her like questionable moral behavior within the organization's culture. It was something that seemed to clearly go against their public mission. Willing to risk unpopularity and not afraid of speaking up, Emily voiced her concerns and eventually left the job. She then moved on to something just as well-compensated that fully embraced her beliefs.

Reaching this state can be scary. After all, going against the group can be a threat to our personal safety. Consider your own mental limits. Perhaps you too were or still are shy; perhaps you get uncomfortable in conflict or have difficulty speaking to perceived authority figures; maybe you freeze when you think your answers (especially the answer, "I don't know") will make you look stupid. For any reason, think of a time when you felt insecure or uncertain. Now think about your body language.

James and Emily, as children, looked down, dropped eye contact, hid behind their mothers, and otherwise made themselves small. Is your body doing something similar? Is your heart rate increasing, or are your back, neck, or shoulders tensing? Do you feel a little queasy? Breathe more shallowly? Restlessly tap your foot? These body sensations may be telltale signs of the thoughts you are currently thinking—what pioneers like Deepak Chopra and Dr. Andrew Weil famously coined as the mind-body connection. Mindset, it turns out, is not only everything to the brain/intelligence, it's everything to the body. And, some say, even the soul.

Stephen W. Porges's groundbreaking polyvagal theory—based on 40 years of data culled from a variety of multidisciplinary studies and supported largely by the work of Bessel van der Kolk with trauma survivors—posits that the vagus nerve operates in various states during every facet of fight-or-flight, including the more rarely identified state of "freeze," when a person shuts down defensively (what our friend James does in both his body and brain in casual social situations). Coining the term "neuroception" to describe how neural circuits judge people and situations as safe or dangerous, Porges theorizes that there are intentional ways to connect physical and mental attunement to grow neuroplasticity among even severely impacted populations like those with schizophrenia and autism. This pioneering work along with Van der Kolk's—who is famously quoted as saying, "The body keeps the score"—traces the psychophysiological roots of that mind-body link between emotions and disease, both with and without overt trauma.

So, when James auto-reverts to broken eye contact and other forms of social detachment with his neighbors, his body may simply be recalling all those childhood years spent as the brunt of shyness jokes.

Fight-or-flight, the survival response born from our earliest brain development processes, provides a simple choice of two different escape options: fighting for our lives or fleeing for safety. Anything that triggers a reminder in our brains or bodies of absolutely anything that could endanger our livelihood will also trigger the neurochemical cascade needed to turn on the fight-or-flight response and transmit it to the heart, lungs, and other body parts via the vagus nerve. Triggers can run the gamut from an unexpected earthquake to a scowl that flits across your supervisor's face during a meeting as you are sharing your brilliant new idea—that then resonates in your subconscious mind as the likelihood you've displeased her and may, therefore, lose your job, or food source.

Using the triune brain model, we can imagine the brain as having three parts: (1) a downstairs basement (often called "the reptilian brain") where the main job is to process all stimuli through a fight-or-flight lens, using emotions to gauge danger; (2) the midbrain, or the ground floor that does the majority of the work learning new ideas and information, then putting them into practice through logic, rote memory, social connections, and building and maintaining relationships via communication; (3) the upstairs, or high brain, that includes the prefrontal cortex—our decision-making portion of the brain and the last to activate in both group and individual human development. Fight-or-flight intentionally shuts down all thinking beyond the "downstairs brain." Why waste time thinking about complexities like how you can cook that attacking animal for dinner when this would only mean distracting yourself and quickly becoming animal food?

Doctors Daniel Siegal and Tina Payne Bryson have written many books on the subjects of neurodevelopment and emotional processing, most notably *The Whole Brain Child*. In this book, they remind parents to "connect through conflict," finding opportunities to teach relationship skills, like seeing the world through others' perspectives. They encourage finding ways to bridge conflict *without losing yourself and your values and views*. It's this kind of perspective on the self and other as validly and equally important to any communal dynamic that places the age-old teaching tactic of shaming on its appropriate shelf to be taken down only when (rarely) necessary: that is, when your actions can cause immediate danger to the greater tribe. As Brené Brown writes, "Shame corrodes the very part of us that believes we are capable of change." As Little

James's brain began to meld shy feelings with shame feelings, his fixed mindset solidified. At least for the moment.

Imagine standing in line for a roller coaster. How do you immediately respond to that? Are you excited at the thrill? Fearful of the perceived torture? Desiring to be a part of the group that loves roller coasters and enjoys the experience even though you are truly frightened out of your wits?

When I ask workshop attendees to share about their relationships with roller coasters, they can typically be split into two camps: those who love roller coasters and can't wait for the ride, and those who are petrified and dread them. I ask one person from each camp to describe what their body feels as they move nearer and nearer the entrance in line. *Both* participants describe the same physical sensations:

- Elevated heart rate
- Shallow breathing
- Energy in the body and a need to move
- Butterflies in the stomach

One camp interprets these body cues as "excitement"; the other as "nervousness." The difference is their brain's perception of these physical sensations—or perhaps their brain's labeling of the sensations as it creates them in tandem with the vagus nerve. Either way, the good news is that *our perceptions can be changed moment by moment.* And when we consciously work together with our bodies, we can practice resilience through acceptance that moves us out of a fixed awareness and into adaptability.

It also moves us into resourcefulness: seeing himself as a capable provider to his family, James's brain kicked into a different mode when his food source/job was threatened, and he suddenly discovered new guides to help him grow, at least in part, in a formerly "stuck" area.

Another interesting point that each roller coaster camp seems to agree on is that *taking deep breaths will calm them down.* It is true that roller coasters are potentially dangerous, and our brains and bodies are alert to this fact. But from yoga practitioners to medical first responders to meditators of every kind, the consensus is the same: breathing deeply sends out a signal—to the brain stem, the vagus nerve, the central nervous system, and probably more—that the worst is over, so we can think rationally, objectively, and fully presently. From women in childbirth to tortured religious saints, we know that this type of profound whole-being connection can transform neurochemistry and suppress pain receptors, even dilate or restrict blood vessels to expedite healing in trauma patients (just ask Judith Acosta and Judith Simon Prager, founders of the verbal first aid lessons for emergency room workers).

As van der Kolk writes in his introduction to Porges' book, "The polyvagal theory legitimates the study of age-old collective and religious practices such as communal chanting, various breathing techniques, and other methods that cause shifts in autonomic state."

In other words, cycling out of fight-or-flight and into higher-level thinking puts the whole being—body, mind, and soul—back online and into the present moment.

Try this exercise:

BMT Index™

Step 1: Think about an uncomfortable experience that makes you feel insecure. This can be speaking in a public setting, meeting a successful person you admire, having to tell someone news they don't want to hear. Think of a situation that is uncomfortable to you. Really put yourself in the moment to conjure up as much detail as you can recall.

Step 2: Ask yourself the following questions: "What does my *body* feel (physical sensations)? What are my *moods*? What are my *thoughts* about it, or what were they in the moment?"

Step 3: Take the time to write down your answers to the above questions. The more detail, the better.

This simple self-assessment in three questions can help you to be present with yourself in your experiences to cycle out of non-life-threatening fight-or-flight, no matter what the trigger. It creates a sort of bridge from the low brain to the high brain, allowing you to become more present yet detached, or *mindful*, and it signals to the reptilian brain that it's okay for the midbrain and prefrontal cortex to come back online.

It's a handy proprietary technique I teach my own communications coaching clients that can be used for everything from simply gaining more insight to thwarting panic attacks, perfectionism, low-level anxiety, OCD-like rumination, and worry. It breaks fight-or-flight down into its moving parts with an understanding that our bodies, moods, and thoughts are interrelated. When we change any piece of the puzzle—through power postures, affirmation statements, positive self-talk, or by engaging in a pleasurable activity such as singing or dancing or deep breathing—we completely disrupt the cycle and our neurochemistry. Over time and repetition, we can replace old negative habits, like breaking eye contact and mumbling greeting, with healthier ones, such as lifting our chins up and squaring our shoulders to give us a natural sense of confidence. Just like Emily did naturally through her mother's encouragement.

From self-talk that self-deprecates to cultural belief systems and axioms that shame, guilt, and otherwise demean, we have, by and large, been a global tribe that coerces individuals to adhere to the group rules and values. But just as the Freudian individuation period lets the toddler run away from their mother with the safety that she'll be there awaiting their return with open arms, so can we, as individuals, use a form of positive disintegration to tear down the socially constructed personalities we may have affixed to concrete labels like "right," "wrong," "happy," "sad," "angry," "shy," "creative," "dependable," "hyper," "focused," "friendly," and more. The reality is that none of these labels is fixed.

We have to remember that not all situations that cause a reaction within us are candidates for our primal fight-or-flight response. If someone is confronted by an undesirable rule within a company, or a culturally unfamiliar custom, for example, fight-or-flight can be triggered. As a result, higher-level thinking shuts down, and we lose our abilities to respond rationally and find solutions that are workable for the diverse group. But as we become ever more socially global, these types of conflicts are bound to occur more readily. When we notice our quickness to negatively judge, criticize, verbally attack, or throw ourselves under the bus with guilty self-talk for not fully going along with the tribe's values, we can lose the opportunity to grow through engaged and respectful conflict.

It may be a relief to realize that encouragement from others, that tribal acceptance that Emily had from birth, is readily available to anyone. Consider, for example, that Dale Carnegie and Napoleon Hill's books have been on US shelves since the 1930s.

Perhaps the greatest mindset shift comes in the form of the answer to that now famous dilemma: Do we live in a friendly or hostile universe?

Ask yourself: Am I okay living like James and growing *only so much*, or am I more like Emily, willing to take risks and find the support I need to grow beyond my current status in life?

You might want to take a deep breath before you answer.

About the Author

Kealah (KEY-la) Parkinson is Coach Kiki, a communications coach who specializes in teaching brain-changing exercises to help clients communicate with ease. From small business owners, sales professionals, and non-profit representatives to teachers, parents, and students, she teaches exercises to help cycle out of fight-or-flight in the moment. Her coaching philosophy is: When you are confident, focused, and authentic with your message, you are a magnet to those you wish to attract. The author of three books and the weekly host of the podcast *Tune In: Radio for Your Mind, Body & Soul*, Kealah is currently writing a daily devotional, pairing mindfulness with mental wellness, *365 Days of Mood Tools*.

Email: ask@coachkiki.com
LinkedIn: linkedin.com/in/kealahparkinson

CHAPTER 19

UNDERSTANDING THE FOUNDATIONS OF LIFE WITH CHINESE MEDICINE

By Robert Prokop, L.Ac
Founder of Wind Gate Wellness, Acupuncturist, Chinese Herbalist
Baltimore, Maryland

As the qi and seasons are regulated, the ten thousand beings are engendered. This is the principle of nature's creation, engenderment, and completion.
–Zhang Jingyue (1563 - 1640 CE)

Did you know your health is connected to the movements of nature? With a history of over 5,000 years, Chinese Medicine can help you understand how your mind, body, and spirit connect to the world around you. You can also use this ancient system to find powerful foods and practices that will benefit each of your major organ systems and boost your health. A few important components of Chinese Medicine are Qi, Yin and Yang, and the Five Elements. Here I'd like to highlight how these work to maintain health and harmony within the human body.

Qi

Qi (pronounced chee) is a foundational component of Chinese Medicine. Often mistranslated as "energy," qi is a much larger concept. It describes the movement, expression, and transformation of all aspects of nature and life. Everything that exists is a manifestation of the movement of qi. The earliest texts from the 3rd and 4th centuries discuss qi as a sort of wind. Think of it as a big, collective oneness that manifests into infinite parts. Each part has its own specific qualities, including yin and yang, and the elements.

Yin and Yang

Picture the popular yin and yang symbol. One part of the symbol is black to represent yin, and the other is white to represent yang. Both are part of the same circle, yet they each have their own directional momentum and way of showing up in the world. They connect: yin creates yang, and yang creates yin. Now, picture the seasons lined up in a similar circle. All have their own frequency, pattern, direction, and individual qualities; but they all exist as a single transformative movement.

When treating disease and illness in Chinese Medicine, practitioners look at the distribution of your qi along the yin/yang spectrum. Yin and yang compliment and balance each other, so if one is excess or deficient, then the other will become out of balance. Imbalance can lead to different states of disharmony and disease. For example, yin is cooling, so a deficiency of it will lead to too much yang, creating heat within the body. Hot and cold are only one example of the many yin/yang spectrums that influence our health. Practitioners will evaluate the energetic balance of each of the five elements in the body.

The Five Elements

The elements are different manifestations of qi. They show up in the world as seasons, colors, flavors, textures, natural phenomena, and more. Each element in Chinese Medicine is of the utmost importance for a balanced life because of their unique gifts, movements, strengths, and weaknesses. Without one element, the whole system falls apart. Qi allows you to integrate the elements from the world around you and from within you. You can transform them into aspects of your physical, emotional, and spiritual life. Learning about the five elements, as they move within you, will help you improve your wellbeing and understand the connection between your body and your emotions. Let's look at the five elements one at a time.

Water

What can we observe from water in nature? It freezes, it evaporates, it forms rivers and contains the majority of life on this planet. One thing about water is that it is rarely not moving. It will always push forward. Water is patient and consistent, with the power to wear away stone over thousands of years. These kinds of energetic qualities are true in people as well. When you look inside yourself to your water element, you'll find deep listening, courage, fear, and your deepest reserves for life. Water is your core of knowledge and pool of wisdom. Ancient people saw the subtle movements of nature and built their lives around this agricultural cycle, so each Chinese element corresponds to a season. Water is connected to winter, with energy like a seed under the ground, lying dormant, and gathering energy for the coming spring. Winter is the most yin time of year as it has the darkest days.

The organs associated with the water element are the kidneys and bladder. Like the seed under the ground, the kidneys contain all the vital energy you need for life. They govern reproductive substances and are said to house your will. The bladder is known for its energy channel which runs down your back. It supports the distribution of qi to all of the organ systems. If these systems are out of balance, symptoms such as knee pain, low back pain, lack of libido, or tinnitus may occur.

Eating specific foods can help balance a particular element and benefit your mind and body. Foods that are dark, black, or purple, such as purple cabbage or black beans, are great for the water element. Organ meats and most foods that come from water are also very balancing. Try incorporating some of these foods into your winter meal planning. Meditation practices and activities like yin yoga or qigong are also very nourishing for the water element by bringing you closer to your primal source.

Wood

From winter, we move to spring: the season of the wood element. In Chinese Medicine, wood is all about rising qi. From this lens, spring starts when qi begins to rise in nature. Where I live in Maryland, that begins in February when the sap begins to rise in trees. The Chinese New Year is on the first day of spring as well. Flowers that were dormant all winter burst forth and grow very quickly, and life begins to rise up to its eventual peak in summer.

Wood in humans is about benevolence, action, decisiveness, and creativity. It connects to a certain type of drive or forward momentum which is translated as anger but is not the same as rage. Wood helps you to manifest actions and plans. It provides you with possibilities and flexibility, and helps you know the pure beauty and power of creation. The wood element helps you see everything in your periphery. It is the new life springing forth from the soil and growing towards the sun, only in people!

The organs associated with wood are the liver and gallbladder. The liver is very important in Chinese Medicine as it houses your ethereal soul and manifests your destiny. It is the embodiment of motivation and decisiveness. When you dream, make plans, or create an itinerary, the liver is behind it. It houses your vision. The gallbladder works in tandem with the vision of the liver. It sees the plans you have laid out and tells you to take action. Both wood organs also have a connection to the tendons and sinews. When the liver or gallbladder get out of balance, it can show up as irritable bowel syndrome, headaches, vision problems, acid reflux, and more. A wood imbalance can also show up as inflexibility (both mentally and physically), frustration, and anger.

To balance the wood element, eat foods that are sour or foods that embody the nature of spring. Asparagus, bamboo shoots, and young greens are all fantastic choices. Stretching exercises will keep your tendons and sinews healthy. Creative outlets like drawing, making music, or journaling allow the wood energy to flow freely without restraint.

Fire

Summer is a time for joy and activity. It connects to fire. Your body can rest more, you don't use as much energy to keep warm, and you can do more outdoor activities. It is the most yang time of year as it has the longest periods of sun. Just like all the elements, fire can show up in a myriad of ways: low burning coals in a fire pit or a raging forest fire. Fire can also spread very quickly, consuming everything within it, but without fuel to combust, fire cannot exist. If you do not tend to your resources in winter, or support your growth in spring, by the time you reach summer, you may not have enough fuel to keep the fire burning.

In people, the fire element is about joy, maturation, laughter, warmth, and partnership. It is your passion and love in the world—the place that connects you to the oneness of the universe. As wood is the rising plant from the seed, fire is the full flourishing bloom. Fire draws you to connect with others and helps you manifest your true self in the world.

Fire has four organ associations: the heart, small intestine, pericardium (heart protector), and triple burner, which is an organ paired with the pericardium and is unique to Chinese Medicine. Different symptoms associated with the fire element include palpitations, insomnia, night terrors, depression, anxiety, and more.

The heart is where your true self lies. On top of its physical responsibilities, it is also in charge of many mental and spiritual activities. When you go to sleep at night your soul resides in the heart, so Chinese Medicine treats many sleep conditions through working with the heart channels. It is considered the emperor of the entire body system, helping your spirit radiate into the world. The small intestine aids communication to the heart, helping you discern what serves you and what doesn't. If you experience trouble with communication or seem to have little or no filter, look to the small intestine.

Fire encompasses so much of your interpersonal communications, intimate experiences, and mental faculties that it also has other systems in place to aid you: the pericardium and triple burner. The pericardium helps the heart open and close to others. While the heart wants to radiate its essence, it may not always be appropriate. The pericardium helps in regulating that process. Finally, the triple burner is the system for distributing heat and fluids throughout the main regions, making sure that the entire kingdom of the body is being properly nurtured.

To maintain a healthy fire element, eat red foods like goji berries, beets, and tomatoes. Bitter foods such as greens also help keep fire under control. Encourage balance within your heart by doing what gives you joy and go easy on yourself.

Earth

The earth element represents late summer when the flowers of the trees have become ripe fruits. There is a relaxed energy and a slow decline in activity. The earth element is at the core of everything, showing up between seasons. The earth holds everything and allows it to exist. It gives plants the ability to root themselves, holds water like a massive bowl, and allows us to live by constantly turning. Earth is the foundation for all life, and its atmosphere encompasses all things, constantly rebuilding and reabsorbing energy.

In people, the earth element is about thoughtfulness, flesh, and the embodied experience of being human. Sweet like fruit, earth is a place of sympathy and care. Internally, it allows your body to break down food into nutrients and disperse them throughout the body. In addition to helping you digest your food, it also helps you digest your emotions. If your earth element is in balance, you'll show up as rooted and secure in yourself. In this balance, you can extend compassion and understanding through empathy and self-reflection. You will work hard, think hard, and know when to relax and reap the benefits of the work you do.

On an organ level, earth is your digestive power. Digestion is all about breaking down, distributing, and integrating the qi of the universe within you. The earth organs, stomach and spleen, are hard workers and support your literal center of being. There is an alchemical beauty that occurs within you every single day; the stomach takes in the outside world and transforms it for you to integrate as part of your body. The spleen distributes qi to the right places, transforms water, and holds you together. In Chinese Medicine, the concept of the spleen includes the pancreatic functions as well. Its primary functions are transformation and transportation. If your spleen becomes deficient, you can become weak, sluggish, drowsy, cold, and have loose stools. This is because the spleen is responsible for transforming food into qi and transforming liquid. If it cannot do either of those jobs to its fullest capacity, you can become damp, deficient, and lack energy.

Taking care of your earth element is important so make sure not to overtax your spleen and stomach. Avoid cold foods such as iced beverages and chilled raw salads (especially in cooler months) to ensure the earth organs don't waste too much energy breaking things down. Also avoid damp producing foods like greasy foods and dairy to ensure a happy spleen. Cooked and easily digestible foods are recommended if you have symptoms of a weak earth element.

Metal

Metal is the element of autumn. In Chinese medicine, metal houses the corporeal soul, or the physical counterpart to your ethereal spirit. Every human's body is like a unique gem or crystal, with their personal soul resonating through it and into the world. Metal is also connected to grief—it is the frequency of autumn, which is when everything returns back into the earth. Inspiration and the art of letting go are also along the frequency of metal. The experience of the metal element can bring with it a profound spaciousness: that moment where you look out in awe at a mountain vista, or when a sad phone call can change your life. It can transform a person like the earth transforms coal into diamonds.

The organs associated with metal are the lungs and large intestine. Qi can be viewed as a gaseous substance or air, and the lungs have a big role in circulating qi around the entire body. They also play a vital role in the body's defenses. When the metal is out of balance, you can experience frequent colds or sinus infections, as well as chronic breathing difficulties. If the lungs are weak, they will have trouble bringing fresh qi into the body and fatigue can set in. From an emotional perspective, the metal element has a lot to do with the idea of self-worth. The large intestine energy helps you physically and emotionally let go of that which does not serve you. Out of balance, it is harder to let go, and you may hold onto things that are not good for you.

Foods that can help support the balance of the metal element are foods that have a dispersing effect and tend to be pungent or spicy. Onions, garlic, radishes, horseradish, and mustard are some examples. You can also balance the metal element through letting go of old habits or old things. Allowing for space and clarity in your external environment can help free up space and clarity in your internal environment.

Integration

As a practitioner who studies and witnesses the Chinese elements in every facet of life, integrating this knowledge has become a way of life for me. I try to balance activities and daily routines to incorporate the gifts different elements offer. When I started the process, it felt like learning to speak a new language, but after incorporating this model into my daily life as a way to look at the world has helped both my physical and mental health. Before I understood the concepts of yin and yang, I used to be very bad about slowing down in the winter and taking the time to cultivate my resources. Although I didn't understand what was happening at the time, this meant my yin energy was very deficient. One way that imbalance showed up for me was that I had frequent mouth ulcers and anxiety. Those symptoms were examples of my fire element not being balanced by my water element. I also used to struggle with digestive issues because I would overtax my spleen by consuming too many damp and raw foods. I have since addressed these health problems by changing my lifestyle and foods I consume. Applying the five-element framework to my life and activities has created many positive changes in my mental and physical health that allow me to live a more full and balanced life.

Applying this framework to life gives me more patience and understanding with the people around me. Some people tend to be more water, while others may be more metal. Everyone has their own levels of comfort and ways they like to manifest. Just like everyone else, I strive for balance, and sometimes things I get offended by come from someone else trying their best in the world, but lacking the understanding that they might be seriously out of balance, which hinders their ability to interact with positive connections with others. Being able to see where others are in their journey has helped me to cultivate a deep listening and empathy, that I'm happy I possess. With this empathy, comes patience and a desire to educate others about the wonderful balance that exists if we just choose to acknowledge the ebbs and flows of qi, yin and yang, and the five elements. These tools have transformed my body and changed my life. It is my sincere hope that you may also enjoy finding a deeper level of well-being within yourself and the world around you through Chinese Medicine.

About the Author

Robert Prokop is a licensed acupuncturist and the founder of Wind Gate Wellness. He received his master's degree in acupuncture in 2016 from Maryland University of Integrative Health and has extensive training in Chinese herbal medicine, Asian bodywork, facial rejuvenation acupuncture, acu-detox, and sports medicine acupuncture. He also attended Naropa University in Boulder, Colorado where he majored in Contemplative Psychology with a focus in health and healing and Buddhist Psychology. He is passionate about the impact of education on wellness goals. Through community workshops in Baltimore and the DC metro area, Robert shares his knowledge and skills to empower individuals to take charge of their own health, thereby creating positive change in their lives and—through a ripple effect—the lives of others.

Email: robert@windgatewellness.com
Website: www.windgatewellness.com

CHAPTER 20
MINDFULNESS, MEDITATION, AND THE BODY

By Wendy Quan
Founder of The Calm Monkey, Workplace
Mindfulness Facilitator Training
Vancouver, British Columbia, Canada

Breathing in, I calm body and mind. Breathing out, I smile.
Dwelling in the present moment I know this is the only moment.
—Thick Nhat Hanh

My Mindful Cancer Story

We're expected to suck it up and deal with a super busy, stressful life, right? Let's face it, unless you decide to give up living in an urban society, you might as well get used to it just like everyone else does. This is how I previously resigned myself to living my life. This was my mindset for living a typical, busy Western lifestyle.

When I look back on my prior lifestyle, I think it was quite typical of many people. I had an office job, a good corporate career climbing the ladder in various contributor and management roles in information technology, human resources, organizational development, and change management. I had a mortgage. I had a family. I had aging parents. I went through a divorce.

I looked after my health. Well, at least I thought I did. I didn't smoke, drink alcohol, or abuse my body. I exercised lightly and stayed fairly active.

My biggest blind spot was my state of being.

What does this mean? I was in a fairly constant state of stressful thinking. I never felt like there was enough time. I was rushing from one thing to the next, feeling the steady pressure of daily life, and admittedly I felt rather proud of myself for being able to juggle work, family, friends, and life's demands successfully.

I didn't realize that although my exterior was fairly calm and cool, my interior didn't match that persona at all. I felt a constant drive to stay busy; otherwise, I felt like I wasn't accomplishing enough. If I saw even one free day on my calendar without bookings, that made me anxious.

And then, I got the proverbial "whack on the side of the head."

In 2010, I received a cancer diagnosis. The diagnosis came just days after my father had a major heart attack. Every artery to his heart was nearly 100 percent blocked, and he was awaiting quadruple bypass surgery. As he didn't expect to survive the surgery, he called the family together at his bedside to say good-bye. During this time, I was also watching over my mom as she needed my support. My daughter was preparing for her high school graduation. Needless to say, it was a monumentally stressful time in my life that I won't forget. I cried in private, and I put on a brave face in front of others.

As a change manager, a profession that helps organizations and people through difficult change, I looked at myself in the mirror and said, *Wendy, you are a change manager, you know that the one thing you have control over is your own reaction to this cancer diagnosis, Dad's heart attack, helping Mom, and ensuring your daughter enjoys her time of graduation.* In that moment, I decided to shift my mindset from the mindset of a powerless victim to the mindset of having strength. But how could I obtain and sustain that strength?

I decided to make my previous dabbling in mindfulness and meditation a regular daily practice. I knew there was plenty of research on the benefits of such practices. I decided not to make any more excuses and just do it.

As I sat in meditation, very quickly, I felt a sense of *being* instead of a sense of overwhelm. I was like a sponge, learning and practicing different types of meditation, and also what it meant to practice mindfulness throughout my day, when I was "off the cushion."

The result was an incredible sense of strength of mind and clarity of thought, which got me through this difficult period of my life. Even today, mindfulness and meditation are very much a part of who I am, and they continue to nourish my emotional and physical healing and sustainment of a healthy, successful body and mind.

I am grateful to say that the cancer diagnosis and my mindfulness and meditation practices changed the trajectory of my life. In 2011, when I returned to my workplace of Pacific Blue Cross in Vancouver, British Columbia, Canada, my co-workers asked me to teach them about mindfulness and meditation. After writing about the benefits my co-workers and my organization were experiencing in a white paper called "Meditation—A Powerful Change Management Tool," a series of astounding events occurred that led me to becoming a pioneer in the workplace mindfulness field. This white paper was awarded the top paper at the 2015 global conference of Association of Change Management Professionals and the peer review committee described it as "ground-breaking." This inspired me to expand my work in the professional workplace mindfulness field.

I am grateful that I have found my life's purpose, which is to
help as many people in the world as possible create a better
experience of life through mindfulness and meditation.

In 2016, I left my corporate career and created The Calm Monkey, which trains and certifies experienced meditators to become skilled mindfulness facilitators and to implement workplace mindfulness with best practices.

The What and Why of Mindfulness and Meditation

Mindfulness and meditation don't have to be complicated. Here is a very simplified explanation of what mindfulness and meditation are, and what the term "mindfulness meditation" means.

Mindfulness is being fully present to what is happening within you and around you, in the present, and with no judgment.

Meditation is the practice of setting aside time in your day to do a meditation. There is an "object" of the meditation—for example, your breath, a mantra, a visualization—and your job is to concentrate and focus on that object. While there are many forms of meditation, it is not all about having a blank mind and does not need to be religious or spiritual. Meditation can include concentration, open awareness, and moving forms like yoga, walking, qi gong, Tai Chi, etc.

Mindfulness meditation is a type of meditation where a person is doing a meditation that keeps them in the present moment. A good example is when someone is meditating on their breath, meaning that breath is the object or focus of the meditation that keeps them in the present moment. A good example of what is not a mindfulness meditation is a guided visualization, where the practitioner is swept away using the imagination into another experience such as visualizing walking along a sandy beach.

For decades, research studies supporting mindfulness and meditation show benefits against an array of both mental and physical conditions. Just to name a few, which seem to be the most discussed benefits, there are the following: reduced anxiety, depression, rumination, stress, chronic pain, blood pressure, and inflammation; and improved immune function, brain function, quality of attention, creativity, and overall resiliency.

It is worthwhile noting that these practices are not always appropriate for everyone. If someone has some residual or unresolved trauma, adverse reactions such as difficult emotions may arise with these practices, so it is important to learn from a qualified instructor, facilitator, or teacher.

Although scientific research is, of course, important, what really mattered to me was my own experience resulting from mindfulness and meditation.

Mindfulness and Meditation Gave Me a Strong Mindset

When I received my cancer diagnosis, I initially was faced with the typical Western medicine route of surgery and pharmaceuticals. I did some of that, but it never felt right to me. Although I didn't have much knowledge of holistic, complementary, and integrative methods, I decided to follow my intuition, and not follow most of what my doctors were telling me to do.

As like most people, mustering up the courage to defy my team of doctors' advice was not easy. Not only that, one needs to have the strength to face all the comments from friends and family. I wasn't rejecting the radiation and drugs as much as wanting to find out what complementary holistic and integrative options were available. I was lucky to find a treasured health advisor who introduced me to the world of credible treatment, testing, supplements, and nutrition.

Mindfulness and meditation gave me the opportunity to tap into my intuition to feel what was the right path for me and gave me the strength to feel at peace with my decisions so that I could do what was best for me.

I am grateful to say that today it has been over ten years since my cancer diagnosis. Through proper nutrition, supplementation, immunotherapy, reducing toxins in my environment, and changing my mindset and state of being through mindfulness and meditation, I proactively test as cancer-free.

Mindfulness and Meditation Improved My Health Issues

Within three weeks of starting a regular daily meditation routine, my blood pressure dropped. I had been on blood pressure medication for over eight years and have been able to discontinue or reduce my blood pressure meditation ever since. I love this example because it is tangible and easily measurable. My eczema improved, as skin health is an indicator of stress. And, my periodic episodes of abdominal pain from gastrointestinal issues disappeared.

Mindfulness and Meditation Nourished My Sense of Belonging

I was raised without religion or spirituality, and as such, felt rather alone. Today, I feel very connected to something bigger than myself and the oneness of us all. Mindfulness and meditation also feed my sense of spirituality.

Mindfulness and Meditation Changed My State of Being

I no longer get caught up in the mind chatter that used to constantly stress me out. I live life with conscious awareness of my thoughts, emotions, behaviors, and intentions. This doesn't mean I live a blissful, constantly happy life, but these practices help me ride the waves of life so much better.

I've often been asked, "Wendy, do you think mindfulness and meditation cured your cancer?" Although I would never say a simple yes to this question, here is what I do say:

- Mindfulness and meditation calmed my mind, which calmed my body, and contributed greatly to shifting my physiology from an environment where disease can grow to one where the body can function in its innate wisdom of self-healing. **If you change the internal environment of your body to a healthier state, then your immune system can do its job and disease cannot flourish. The mind-body connection is not something to be ignored.**

- Mindfulness and meditation changed my state of being from being in a constant state of stressful thinking to one of self-awareness, strong intention, clarity of mind, healthy perspectives, and strength of mind to live life in a state of conscious awareness rather than in stressful autopilot.

- To create a healthy body is a multi-factorial endeavor that includes meditation, but you also need to create a healthy state of being, nourishing yourself with whole foods, good quality sleep, reducing toxins, breathing properly, and exercising sufficiently.

How Mindfulness and Meditation Contribute to a Healthy Body

Particular evidence that has caught my attention regarding how mindfulness and/or meditation relate/s to a healthy body include:

- Mind-body practices that elicit the relaxation response have been used for millennia to prevent and treat disease. In the 1970s, Dr. Herbert Benson, a professor at Harvard Medical School, coined the term "relaxation response," identifying it as the common, functional attribute of transcendental meditation, yoga, and other forms of meditation. The relaxation response is the opposite of the body's adrenaline-charged "fight-or-flight" response. Benson insisted that the mind plays a critical role in the body's health and disease states.

- Dr. Jeffery Dusek proved that the relaxation response changes which genes are activated in the blood. Meditation turns on counter-stress genes and turns off stress genes.

- Dr. Daniel Goleman and Dr. Richard J. Davidson have done admirable research as presented in their book *Altered Traits* that shows what meditation can do for the brain, the body, and the mind.

- Dr. Lissa Rankin's book *Mind Over Medicine* lists meditation as one of many things needed for self-healing of the body.

One particular resource I would like to highlight is Dr. Joe Dispenza, a renowned teacher and researcher. He has helped many people worldwide use the power of meditation and neuroplasticity to rewire their brains to produce significant change in their lives. Many have used his teachings to heal physical and emotional issues. I learned of Dr. Dispenza in 2012 from a friend who has multiple sclerosis and was using a wheelchair about half the time. After practicing Dr. Dispenza's meditation techniques, she was able to live life without her wheelchair. That sparked me to take all of Dr. Dispenza's workshops, where I met many people who have been helped, including a quadriplegic who can now sit up and feed himself. I believe that his method is a significant component of my healing from cancer and continues to help sustain my good health.

Simple Techniques to Calm the Mind and the Body

Everyone's experience with mindfulness and meditation is unique. Even from one meditation session to the next, a person might experience very different results or no results at all. The spectrum of benefits varies greatly; however, the first benefit most people notice is a sense of relaxation and calm.

Four Attitudes for Successful Meditation

I teach four attitudes to beginner and experienced meditators alike. These are wildly successful, and they help dispel the myths and contribute to a more successful and sustained mindfulness and meditation practice.

1. **Have No Expectations.** I like to say, "If you don't have any expectations, you can't get frustrated." Don't expect a blank, empty mind. Your human mind will naturally wander. You want to notice when the wandering is occurring, and then gently bring your focus back to your meditation.
2. **Have No Judgment.** Don't judge yourself or your meditation practice. Regard each meditation as a unique experience, and don't judge your experiences against others.
3. **Have a Beginner's Mind.** Go into each session with a freshness, not forcing anything in particular to happen, even if you are an experienced meditator.

4. **Be an Observer.** Be a curious witness to what happens during your meditation. Notice how you are concentrating, when your mind wanders, and how you feel physically and emotionally during and after the session.

Simple Mindful Breathing

There are countless types of meditation practices, but if you are unfamiliar with mindfulness and meditation, perhaps the easiest thing to start with is to sit quietly where you won't be disturbed or feel self-conscious, and do this simple breathing technique.

1. Sitting in a chair, sit up tall using your back muscles, but still be relaxed. Sitting tall will allow you to breath better and more comfortably. Have both feet flat on the floor.
2. If you feel comfortable closing your eyes, please do so, but also know that you may keep your eyes slightly open with a soft, unfocused gaze in front of you, if you wish.
3. Through your nose, inhale slowly and—still sitting relaxed—count silently to yourself, "One, two, three, four, five." Then exhale and count silently, "One, two, three, four, five." Keep repeating. The idea is to have a soft, relaxed rhythmic breathing cadence. Observe all that is going on in your body as you do this—the subtle physical movements, the air flowing in and out of your nostrils, the thoughts that appear, etc.
4. Remember the four attitudes of having no expectations, no judgments, a beginner's mind, and being an observer.
5. If and when you find that you have lost count, simply restart the breathing with counting again. No judgment. No expectations.

After you perform your breathing meditation for a few minutes, check in with yourself and see how you feel. There is no right or wrong way to feel, but this may invoke the relaxation response in your body. A common benefit of a rhythmic breathing meditation is a feeling of calm in your mind and body.

Actionable Advice and Parting Words

1. Learn more about mindfulness and meditation. There are countless ways to learn through apps, books, and online sessions. However, it is best to learn live from a qualified instructor, facilitator, or teacher, so you can have dialogue and ask lots of questions.
2. Make time. I often hear the excuse, "I don't have time to meditate". The reality is, everyone has time to meditate if they choose to do so. A meditation session may be two minutes or an hour long; it's up to you. Instead of spending ten minutes checking social media or watching a show, meditate for an improved state of being, amongst all the many other benefits you may get.

It took a frightening cancer diagnosis for me to wake up to a more mindful, enjoyable life. You've seen my story of how my state of being dramatically shifted through practicing mindfulness and meditation. It was through consciousness self-awareness and taking a different perspective on how I was living my life that led to my body's healing and made me a much happier person. Mindfulness and meditation have changed my state of being and created a better experience of life. I wish the same outcome for you.

Whether you are struggling with stress or a health issue, or if you just want to see how much more free your mind and body can feel, I encourage you to explore meditation and mindfulness as a way to help you live in your very own successful body.

About the Author

Wendy Quan, founder of The Calm Monkey, is an innovator and industry leader in mindfulness meditation facilitator training and certification. She is also a pioneer in combining change management with mindfulness to help people through difficult change, and she is a professional speaker.

As a certified organizational change manager, Wendy's award-winning, published white paper "Meditation—A Powerful Change Management Tool" presents the case study of how she achieved 25 percent of Pacific Blue Cross' employees attending mindfulness sessions and boosted change resiliency through a major transformation.

With her corporate management background in human resources, information technology, organizational development, and change management, together with her personal mindfulness meditation experience through cancer, she is one of the leading authorities for workplace mindfulness. She has been recognized as a pioneer by the Greater Good Science Center of the University of California, Berkeley, and the global Association of Change Management Professionals and Mindful Leader.

Wendy's clients have included Google, the government of Dubai, Genentech, Citrix, U.S. National Park Service, Rich Products, and hundreds of individuals trained as facilitators worldwide. Her cancer journey led to her life's purpose: "To help people create a better experience of life through mindfulness meditation." The mission of The Calm Monkey is "creating a mindful world, together." To learn more about Wendy and The Calm Monkey, reach out to her directly.

Email: Wendy@TheCalmMonkey.com
Website(s): https://www.thecalmmonkey.com/
https://www.linkedin.com/in/wendyquan/
https://www.facebook.com/TheCalmMonkeyCo

CHAPTER 21

YOUR LIFE, YOUR POTENTIAL, YOUR REVOLUTION

By Jay Quarmby
Personal Trainer, Lifestyle Coach
Toronto, Canada

A goal is not always meant to be reached, it often
serves simply as something to aim at.
—Bruce Lee

Your physical health affects every single aspect of your life. It's connected to the way you think, the way you view yourself, the way others view you, and how you feel emotionally. Everything in your life is affected by your health and fitness.

Before you read another sentence, bookmark this chapter because you're going to want to come back to it as a reference. I'm going to share five critical steps required to achieve the level of health and fitness you've always dreamed of. The reason most people continuously jump on and fall off the wellness wagon is because they usually only focus on two or three of these steps, or they follow them in the wrong order. Unless you follow these steps in sequence when attempting to transform your life, I can't guarantee you won't be back at your starting point six months later. Because of its fundamental value, I'm going to focus primarily on step one.

Before we get into the practical stuff, I have one incredibly important point I must impart to you: having the right MINDSET must come first. It's so important I must repeat this: **having the right MINDSET must come before anything else.** Forget about trying to implement any of the other amazing fitness and nutrition strategies outlined in this book without mindset. They are useless to you if you don't focus on having the right mindset in place first.

To really push yourself to your next level of health and fitness, I want you to think about the term, *a personal revolution.* Whether you've never attempted to add health and fitness to your life before, or you've been working at it for a long time, but you've plateaued and want to achieve more, you need to approach your transformation under the mindset of "a personal revolution." The word "revolution" means a "forcible overthrow of a government or social order, in favor of a new system, or a drastic political or social change that usually occurs relatively quickly." When it comes to a personal revolution, it's the same idea: we need to overthrow our life, the "government" that is running our daily routine, our choices, our habits. We need a new system!

When you think of different revolutions throughout history, they generally occurred because citizens were so unhappy that they got to a breaking point; they rose up and made a change. We can also get to that same point in our lives where we have just had enough, and we need to change NOW.

So, do you want to feel good, look great, live better, and optimize your health and fitness? If so, take action now and put everything you've got into it. This is the start of a revolution; you're taking over!

The 5-Step Process to Achieving a Personal Revolution.

- Step 1: **Clarity**—figure out your who, what, why, how
- Step 2: **Measurement**—when you track it, you can improve it
- Step 3: **Discipline**—create positive habits and maintain them
- Step 4: **Nutrition**—eat healthily. Live well. Feel great
- Step 5: **Exercise**—movement is the foundation of life

I want you to notice something important here. Notice that **nutrition** and **exercise** are the last two steps, not the first. This is critical. This is where most people get it wrong. Ninety-nine percent of people start at these two steps, usually by joining a gym, getting a trainer, maybe starting a new diet plan at the same time. This will give you short-term success, and although you might even last a couple of years focusing on just these two things, it only takes one slight disruption in your life, like moving house, changing jobs, personal life stress, or any slight change to your routine, and the house of fitness and nutrition cards comes tumbling down.

Moving or changing jobs are perfect examples. Last time you moved or changed jobs, how was your health and routine affected? Did you fall off the wagon? How long did it take to get back to a routine?

Step 1: Clarity

Until you're crystal clear in your mind why you want to live better and why you want to be fit and healthy, you aren't going to have permanent life-changing results. You need to find reasons so deep and so personal that no excuse or life disruption is good enough to keep you from your workout or dissuade you from staying on track with your personal health goals. To better explain this concept, I ask my clients a simple question, "Why do you go to work every day? Surely you don't enjoy doing that all the time." Everyone can give me a list of reasons why going to work every day is important to them. Their answers include:

- *I want to provide for my family.*
- *I have a mortgage I have to pay.*
- *I want money to travel.*
- *I need to be able to buy clothes and groceries.*
  The list goes on and on.

I follow this up by asking the question, "Why do you think I focus on my health and fitness every day? I don't enjoy doing that all the time."
My reasons are:

- *I want to live longer to be around my family.*
- *I want to minimize my chances to get sick or injured.*
- *I want to optimize my capacity to work harder since I'm fit and healthy.*
- *I want people to respect me more for my discipline.*
- *I want to be able to keep up with my children.*
- *I want to be physically attractive to my partner.*
  The list goes on and on.

Can you see now that I consider my health and fitness to be as important to me as you consider your career and job to be to you? This doesn't mean that I don't prioritize my career. I've been an entrepreneur my whole life, working as hard as anyone else. I've spent many years working from 6 am to 8 pm, five to six days a week. I also understand that to be the best version of myself, especially in my career, I need to prioritize my health and fitness first.

Now let's do a short exercise. For it to work, I need you to be willing to dig deep and uncover some potential pain and discomfort in order to gain the clarity and mindset you need to break through the cycle you've been on and achieve a permanent dedication to a new, healthier, better version of you.

Take my list of reasons why I prioritize my health and fitness, and write down the reverse of them, using "If ... then" sentences. For example:

- *If I don't prioritize my health and fitness, I'm less likely to live longer.*
- *If I don't prioritize my health and fitness, I'm more likely to get sick or injured.*
- *If I don't prioritize my health and fitness, my capacity to work harder will decline.*
- *If I don't prioritize my health and fitness, ...*

Continue down the list and start adding some of your own reasons. I want you to make your list so long that when you read it, it frightens you. The thought of not looking after yourself doesn't justify the outcomes you can see on that list. Just like the thought of "If I don't go to work and make money, I won't be able to pay my mortgage" makes you get out of bed and go to work, the thought of, "If I don't prioritize my health and fitness, I won't be around as long as I can for my family" should be enough to make you get out of bed and do a workout.

I suggest spending some time focusing on this negative list until the severity of it sinks in, and then I want you to rewrite the opposite of all these negative outcomes into a new list of positive outcomes. Keep this list on your phone, on the fridge, or on the back of the bathroom door, so that you are constantly reminded of all the positive things you are gaining by sticking to a health and fitness routine. This list will help you think about how amazing your life will be by simply prioritizing your health and fitness. You should be feeling not only positive but determined not to fall off the wagon because now you know the negative impact if you don't stay focused.

Now that you have clarity on why you need and want to be healthy and fit, the next exercise is to envision what it is you actually want to achieve by being healthy and fit. What does the healthy, fit version of yourself look like? If you're now prioritizing your health and fitness, then what do you want to get out of that. Let's create some tangible goals to work towards.

- Do you want to be strong and muscular?
- Do you want to be lean, fit, and flexible?
- Do you want to be able to play tennis well into your older years?
- Do you want to be able to fit into a dress two sizes smaller?

What do you want? Think big, think outrageous, think about what would really feel like a massive win for you. Write it down. This is now what you genuinely want for yourself; this is now your health and fitness goal. What amazing things do you want for yourself now? I want to know!

Let me explain what we have just done and why this is so powerful. I don't want you turning another page until you really get this.

By writing down the negative list of what will happen if you don't prioritize your health and fitness, we have created enough purpose and conviction within you to show that it is really worth focusing on over the long term, i.e., the rest of your life. Then, by stacking on a list of goals to work towards, you not only have the long-term reasons, you now have a list of short-term reasons why you're doing this.

When I go to the gym I'm thinking, "I need to work out so that I keep my energy levels up and I'll stay healthy." I'm also thinking, "I need to work out so that I continue to lose body fat since it's nearly summer, and I'm going to be taking my shirt off." My long-term goal is to keep my energy high and stay healthy, and my short-term goal is to reduce my body fat so that I have a six-pack visible when I take my shirt off in the sun. The combination of long- and short-term goals has kept me motivated and focused on my health and fitness for over 20 years now.

The next exercise I want you to work through is figuring out exactly how you're going to achieve the long- and short-term goals you have now discovered are important to you. If running your first 5K race is one of your goals, how are you going to do that? Are you just going to turn up at the starting line and run the 5K race when you've never run before? I doubt it.

This is where MINDSET comes back into play again. You need to take ownership of your goals and decide that YOU are going to work towards them; no one else can achieve them but you. Of course, you can and should get help, but your trainer or coach can't run the 5K race for you, you actually have to do it.

I want you to look at your list of long- and short-term goals and create a game plan of how you are going to achieve them. I want this list to be an actionable, step-by-step account of everything you plan to do. What is the very first step you are going to take? For instance, your first step might be one these:

- **Step 1** Sit down and go through the exercises Jay has laid out in this chapter, so I have clarity on why my health and fitness are important to me and what my goals are.
- **Step 1** Ask my network for a recommendation for a personal trainer because I don't know how to work out and I need help.
- **Step 1** Buy a pair of running shoes because I want to run a 5K race, and I don't own any.

Your second step might be one of these:

- **Step 2** Start implementing one of the other strategies that I connected with in this book, I'm going to use that to help me achieve my short-term goal of losing weight.
- **Step 2** Call three of the personal trainers I was recommended and book a consultation to figure out which one I want to work with.
- **Step 2** Find a "Learn to Run" class in my area and sign up.

Your third step might be:

- **Step 3** (You write it in!)

Keep going for as long as you can, and remember, the more steps you have, the easier it is to simply work your way down the list and stay laser focused on what you want to achieve. Just follow your list of steps, no guesswork, no uncertainty, it's all laid out there on the paper. And guess what? you made that list, you took ownership of your health and fitness, not me, not anyone else. You did it.

Even the act of completing the list is something to celebrate. If you haven't made your list yet, make a goal to finish it before the end of today.

Once you've gone through these clarity exercises you have officially gone through step one of the five-step process to achieving a personal revolution. Once the first step is completed, you're not done, but the other four steps will easily fall into place for you.

Step 2: Measurement

Simply measure and track your results based on what your goals are now. If your goal is to lose weight, then measure your weight loss, and select a specific weight you want to be at, so you can track your progress. If your goal is to run a 5K race, then set markers for your progress, for example, one mile by the end of the first week, two miles by the end of the month, three miles by the end of the third month, etc. Track each week how far you run until you can comfortably run five kilometers. If you don't track the distance, how will you know how far you've run? And, reaching milestones helps keep you engaged and excited.

Step 3: Discipline

Now that you have your game plan and step-by-step plan of how you're going to achieve your goals, you need the discipline to keep working your way through the list. The discipline comes through taking action and creating habits that align with achieving your goals. If your goal is to lose weight, then you use discipline to make sure you aren't overindulging on food and alcohol. If your goal is to run a 5K, then become disciplined to practice running three times per week.

Step 4: Nutrition

Whatever your goals are, you can find a nutrition and diet plan that will work for you. If you want to lose weight, you use a weight loss plan. If you want to run a 5K, you can find a nutrition plan that runners use, and you follow that. Get excited about the positive changes that will occur as you decide on the best nutrition plan for yourself.

Step 5: Exercise

Exactly the same as nutrition, whatever your goals are, find a workout and exercise plan that will align with your goals. If you want to lose weight, focus on exercise that will burn calories and keep you in a fat-burning state. If you want to run a 5K, then obviously your exercise plan is going to include a lot of running.

I hope you can see that until you have crystal clear vision around why you're trying to be healthy and fit, it's going to be extremely difficult to stay focused on and dedicated to an exercise plan or a diet. How can you pick and stick with a diet or workout routine if you don't know exactly why you want to be healthy and fit in the first place?

Whether you're just embarking on the journey of health and fitness for the first time, or you're a veteran of the game, these clarity exercises will help you to achieve the body you want and to achieve goals in your personal life you've only previously imagined. I return to the five steps again and again as a powerful tool to reset my goals and launch myself towards my next personal fitness endeavor. As my body changes, I level up with a new set of goals.

Now it's your turn … It's your life, it's your potential, it's *your* Personal Revolution.

About the Author

Jay Quarmby is a personal trainer, lifestyle coach, fitness instructor, and entrepreneur. His passion for transformational experiences comes from his own personal revolutions. From packing his bags and moving across the globe from Sydney to Toronto, to competing in natural bodybuilding and physique shows, these life-changing experiences have shown him the importance of self-discovery and self-discipline. Jay runs a six-month life transformation program that helps overworked executives restore balance to their life through health and fitness optimization while maintaining their high-functioning careers.

If you would like to achieve your own personal revolution, head over to Jay's website and grab a copy of his book *Your Personal Revolution—Five Steps to Taking back Control of your Health & Fitness.* This actionable book will take you step by step in detail through his five-step process.

Jay loves video games, working out, his wife Lucy, traveling the world, and deep debates with friends, although not necessarily in that order.

Email: jay@thepersonalrevolution.com
Website: www.thepersonalrevolution.com
Instagram @thepersonalrevolution

CHAPTER 22
THE TOTAL PACKAGE

By James Rizzo
Owner of Fitness Scientist LLC
New York, New York

Strength does not come from winning. Your struggles develop your strengths.
When you go through hardships and decide not to surrender, that is strength.
—Arnold Schwarzenegger

The phrase "total package" has been used to describe men and women who seem to have it all. To be a total package means you're on a high level—physically, mentally, emotionally, and spiritually. In order to be the **total package**, you need to consider your packaging, which, of course, includes your physical body itself as well as other elements, all of which we'll go into in this chapter.

The first component of the total package to consider is the physical body, which impacts both your physical exterior as well as your overall health. Regular physical exercise is one of the most important things people can do to improve their appearance and overall health. Moving more and sitting less have tremendous benefits to everyone, regardless of age, sex, race, ethnicity, or current fitness level.

People who have an envious physique are the ones who put in the work, plain and simple. Professional athletes are an example. It takes incredible discipline, consistency, and will power to achieve top-level goals. The physical specimen is like a well-oiled machine. It needs constant maintenance in order to operate at peak performance. I describe this to my clients as being "garage kept." By using this metaphor, they clearly understand if it comes down to the choice of leaving a car on the street or safely in a garage, the answer should be obvious. The more valuable the car, the more likely the owner will want to keep it inside. I reiterate that we should treat our body with the same respect by putting our health first.

Another thing I often remind clients is the idea, "If you don't use it, you lose it." This is particularly important in prolonged exercise to maximize your results. I try to envision myself in the future and visualize exactly what I want to look like and who I want to be, and that's what motivates me to keep pushing forward.

A specific type of fitness that I specialize in with my clients is strength training. Sadly, only 17 percent of Americans incorporate strength training into their workouts. Yet, the benefits are priceless. The main benefits of strength training on the body are an increase in metabolism which helps you to lose weight and acquire lean muscle mass. Strength training helps fight infectious diseases by boosting your immune system. Bone density deteriorates as we get older and is a major problem for a large population of people who suffer from osteoporosis and osteopenia. These conditions are oftentimes hereditary, which can cause bones to become brittle and fragile from loss of tissue, typically as a result of hormonal changes, or a calcium or vitamin deficiency. Strength training is a perfect way to counteract these ailments.

Strength training and exercise aren't simply for aiding you in terms of your appearance and physical health. They also give you robust mental health, another critical component in the total package.

During trying times, exercise can provide an indispensable mental-health support for many of us. Among generally healthy but sedentary adults, exercise lowers levels of depression, hostility, and other negative feelings. The mood benefits of exercise can linger for weeks after people stop working out, offering another compelling reason for us to keep moving, whenever and wherever we still can, especially during difficult times. Regular exercise substantially reduces risks for clinical depression among people with a genetic predisposition to the condition and helps treat serious depression. Likewise, daily exercise often alleviates the severity of anxiety disorders.

My wife, who is an attending psychiatrist in New York, diagnoses and treats mental illness. Exercise has been a staple in her life, physically and mentally. It clears her mind of any negativity she normally encounters during her rigorous work environment, and she encourages patients to use exercise in their routines as another tool in dealing with mental illnesses as well.

According to the *Translational Sports Medicine Journal*, between two minutes and one hour of aerobic exercise such as running, walking, or cycling improves learning and memory function in young adults. Exercise at moderate to high intensity, even for just 120 seconds, improves learning, memory, planning, problem-solving, concentration, and verbal fluency. And these positive effects can last up to two hours.

In order to maintain discipline and consistency, it is best to have complete control over your emotions. Too many of us, including me, get used to dwelling on uncontrollable situations, work/personal problems, etc., instead of focusing on what we can control. Emotionally healthy people still feel stress, anger, and sadness, but they know how to channel their negative feelings to live a better life. Exercise helps us with emotional regulation and channeling negative feelings.

Along with maintaining vigorous physical and mental health, another key component of the total package is having a spiritual center—believing in yourself is made so much easier when you have faith in all areas of life. I acquired my strong family values and morals from my parents who have always embraced their Italian heritage and the Catholic faith. My family and I believe in going to church on Sunday and saying grace before meals. I make it a point to ask God for forgiveness, pray for others, and allow Him to pave the correct path for me. I don't have all the answers; I still don't understand why bad things happen to good people, but if you do what is right, not what is easy, you will know what success means.

I'm a big believer in karma, good and bad, and I've seen some really high highs and some really low lows, but I learned from every experience, including a short, forced encounter with homelessness after suddenly losing everything I had. I now tell anyone going through hardship—*if you've seen the worst, then you can appreciate the best.*

One of the main reasons I chose fitness as my profession is the ability to give someone something they've never experienced before … empowerment! The process of becoming stronger and more confident to take control of your life is truly rewarding. Nothing keeps a person more motivated than real results. I get a sense of self-worth from my clients' dedication. They appreciate me, and I appreciate them. Luckily, my job never feels like work because the rapport I share with my clients is genuine. I continually check in to see how they're feeling. If necessary, it is imperative to modify the workout because having precise form will reduce discomfort and is essential to their well-being. Through witnessing so many people transform through a well-planned exercise regimen, I hold that *daily exercise and maintenance are the closest thing you can get to the fountain of youth.*

In any difficult situation, it is important to adapt to the needs of others. During the height of the 2020 coronavirus pandemic, I had to move my in-person training business online, but I strongly believe that for every negative action, there's a positive reaction. My innovative abilities were constantly challenged by minimal resources. Many of my clients had little to no equipment to work with. My solution: I incorporated more "functional training" into my clients' workout routines. Performing movements such as step-ups, stability, deadlifts, and squats will not only build more core muscles and strength, but they are essential to everyday life. This learning experience eventually made me excel at virtual training. As a result, my clients remain happy and healthy. The negative situation turned into a positive outcome.

The qualities that have had the most impact on my success as a fitness scientist are building a good reputation, maintaining a positive attitude, and staying personable, and these are all qualities which I consider indispensable in having the total package. During my youth, my grandfather spoke of reputation as being the most important attribute a person can possess. Reputation shapes how people behave, what people buy, how they think, and why people act the way they do. A good reputation provides better clients and more trust. I made plenty of mistakes in life, but I use those mistakes to fail forward. Your reputation is the underlying factor any person or business will consider first.

A person's attitude will make or break a company, a church, or a home. One of my favorite quotes is "Life is ten percent what happens to you and 90 percent how you react to it." We are truly in charge of our attitudes and our ultimate destiny. Having an excellent attitude is a personal choice. You can either beat yourself up or refuse to surrender to negativity. It can take many years to perfect this. Emotional weakness won't change a thing, and typically it fuels disappointment. Perfecting a positive attitude will improve your exercise plan as well as your business and personal relationships tenfold.

A perfect example of a positive attitude is my mother, who was recently diagnosed with Parkinson's disease. She is someone who refuses to surrender. When she first learned of her diagnosis, she struggled to accept it. It's hard for anyone to understand how your neurological functions will be compromised because of a dopamine deficiency. But now, she uses daily exercise to combat her stiffness and improve her mobility. Walking, cycling, and training with her son—me—has become her weekly routine. As a result, she has more energy, flexibility, and a better acceptance of her limitations.

Being personable is the last factor to consider in the total package that I'll discuss. Anyone can look the part but if they're arrogant or dishonest, their ego deteriorates everything else about them. I try to be the person everyone can count on to get the fitness results they want, but I also try to lead with humility. I believe these qualities often lay the foundation for success.

I knew at a very young age that my calling was to teach and lead others. With over 20 years' experience in the fitness industry, I started training clients in commercial gyms such as Bally Total Fitness, World Gym, Equinox, Boom Fitness, and David Barton. After I developed enough experience working in various training environments, I knew I had the potential to build my own brand and establish myself in the fitness community. For the past 14 years, I've worked as a private personal trainer, and I've had the opportunity to work with many wonderful individuals who have transformed their lives. I'm passionate not only about transforming my clients, but I'm also passionate about challenging myself and learning something new every day. The fitness industry has been an amazing catalyst for me because it has helped me get my body to a healthy state that I can be proud of, and it has allowed me to give back and help others on their own fitness journeys. Through training others, my purpose is beyond myself, and that means a lot to me.

About the Author

James Rizzo was raised in Wilmington, Delaware. His parents sent him to parochial schools and insisted his education be done in a private setting. He is very proud of his parents and his loyalty to them is expressed with the love and respect they share. James's childhood was different from most because of his strict upbringing without siblings. He was extremely shy and was bullied because of his appearance of being tall and lanky with glasses. He became very defensive and couldn't rely on others because of his lack of trust, so he needed to stand on his own. Over time, James came to know himself and what he needed to do to develop the confidence he yearned for. He took up exercise as a hobby at 11 years old only to build his body as a means to construct self-confidence and respect from others. He dedicated his extracurricular activities to develop a strong core, both physically and emotionally, and realized he was in charge of his future. By immersing himself in fitness, his attitude and aspirations improved more and more. James used bodybuilding to develop the confidence he needed to earn respect from others, which drives him to excel today. He can honestly say he's never been stronger than he is now, and he owes it all to the grace of God, respect for himself, and the love and support from his wife and parents.

Email: jamesjrizzo@gmail.com
Website: www.fitnessscientist.com

CHAPTER 23
YOUR MIND CONTROLS YOUR SUCCESS

By Jeanette Ruiz
Mind, Body & Spirit Coach, Keynote Speaker
New York, New York

I often say, "We must understand that the past is already gone, and the future is now. Transformation begins ... now!" Right now is the moment that our transformation must begin. Our beliefs, thoughts, and fears have all been embedded in our being by generational beliefs and by everything else under the sun that has impacted our lives. When we refuse to care about what others say and think of us, we grow. We begin to no longer care if we are laughed at when we fall or stumble, knowing that we can dust ourselves off, get up, and try over again. So, let us consider the following questions and reflect upon them for a moment:

- When do you want to start performing with your greatest potential to achieve your fitness goals?
- When do you want to start to listen to your unique body? (We do not have the same blueprint as others, making each of us completely different, both in chemical and molecular structures.)

- When do you want to start fueling yourself both physically and mentally to be transformed?
- When do you want to realize that, as time changes, so does your thinking and your awareness of your body's greatest potential?

The time is now. You can succeed in weight loss and body transformation when you can create and recreate performance achievements. It always comes down to the three primary aspects of success: mindset, emotions, and grit. In understanding how our mindset, emotions, and grit balance each other out, we gain a better understanding of how to achieve our goals in a successful and attainable manner. First, in this chapter, we'll look into the roles of mindset, emotions, and grit, and after that we'll look at how our subconscious and conscious minds come into play in our quest to achieve optimal mental and physical transformation right now.

Mindset, Emotions, and Grit

Mindset—when we allow our mind to create fear, anxiety, and self-doubt, we keep ourselves from succeeding, and we miss out on so many opportunities. These obstacles are emotions that we allow to well up within us, emotions that we have felt in the past and that we are carrying tucked away in our mind, constantly dictating some of our decisions. We do not realize that they emerge from our memory every time we are confronted with the same or a similar situation.

Emotions—harmful emotions such as fear, anxiety, and self-doubt can hold us back from our dreams, from creating our ideal routines, and from reprogramming ourselves for success. Emotions come from habits that we created surrounding various situations that impacted our mind. There are habits that we put in place as triggers to steer us from things that are unfamiliar to our being. Emotions will bring back memories that will stunt our growth. All our thoughts and perceptions are created in our minds and in our memories that get jumbled up with all our decisions. Whether true or false, right or wrong, good or bad, our experiences tend to absorb into our thought patterns. This is where mindset, grit, and everything else come together.

We have to start erasing the canvas that has been placed before us and start rewriting who we are. We have to start seeing ourselves as the vision that our imagination has allowed us to desire, to want, to dream of, in terms of our physique, confidence, and personality. It is time to stop worrying about how we are perceived and start embracing who we are, how far we have come, and how far we are going to take our potential.

Grit—within the concept of grit lies the moment of truth to the success level that we are looking to achieve. The moment where we know what we want and how much we are willing to sacrifice to achieve it. Everything begins with our passion, how hungry we are to obtain that success and how much effort we'll put into living it, thinking it, and breathing it into existence. We can see it in our mind during the meditative moments when we are with ourselves in our thoughts. We can have many things that excite our passion that can seem to go together, working towards our primary goal or desire, but it's only one specific thing that will stand out above the rest. That is our passion, the one thing we focus on that gives us all the energy to fight until we obtain a goal, no matter the obstacles we are confronted with.

When we find our passion, we will seek information to build on it. Then we will share our findings and accomplishments with others. The willingness to chase that passion at all costs comes from our inner level of grit, even if there is no way to be sure we will get where we want to be. We will get right back on track no matter how many times this cycle is repeated. Every decision we make will be focused on dedicating a great amount of our time to this passion, which may be our fitness and weight loss plan. Once we've reached that potential, our mind will shift and set a new standard for our next level. When we find our grit for pursuing our passion, we are unstoppable.

The Role of Our Subconscious Mind

Our thinking has the power to work for or against us. Our conscious and subconscious minds play a huge role in the choices we make, primarily affecting our execution of things we want to do, our decisions, and our viewpoints.

Our subconscious mind is constantly working with what is familiar to us, from our birth until our expiration on this earth. These habits and programs that have been embedded in our mind hold all our thoughts and memories. They have been created by situations we have endured throughout our lives, whether traumatic from verbal, emotional, or physical abuse, from injuries and disappointments, or through our positive memories of happiness and accomplishments throughout life. Different circumstances may have occurred even during a competition, test, or challenge, or get brought upon us by other people at home, work, the gym, etc.

Events that we hold in our subconscious mind create the framework of both our fight-or-flight mechanism and our logical thinking. These thoughts, memories, and habits have been programming us since our very first breath. They have created memory patterns for situations and confrontations and have kept us from unlocking our full potential. This is where all our habits—the good, the bad, and the ugly—come from. They hold our why. Why are we who we are? Why do we act, think, do, and not do? Things we decide to do or not do, at times, keep us from evolving into someone more amazing, and more powerful than we currently are.

Our subconscious mind holds the key to our mental and physical trans-formation. When we tap into the "why," then and only then will we begin to understand that we need to rewire our brains and break the program that has been installed in us since our early years. It is our subconscious mind that holds the blueprint to our life's ups and downs. However, if we decide to stick with our subconscious mind, then we'll only be functioning via an emotional state from the past, the hardwiring that was embedded in our thinking.

To overcome living and thinking in the subconscious, we need to rewire all those programs. From the moment we challenge ourselves to change, we rewire our programmed brain. The time to start is now. If procrastinating is the problem, we'll be stuck in a whole other loop of starting and stopping, and we'll never reach our true self. It might seem challenging, but when we imagine our new reality, we will desire change. It takes repetition and consistency to implant change in order to start seeing progress.

Tapping into Our Subconscious Mind

There are many ways to reprogram our subconscious mind. One way is to learn to tap into self or guided hypnosis. It isn't difficult. After all, we take our brain into a hypnotic state while we are asleep. During this time, our subconscious mind is stepping forward and our conscious mind is stepping back. This is where brains are hardwired. Anyone can also obtain this state while awake with the help of a hypnotherapist, through meditation, or simply by listening to or speaking daily affirmations.

Athletes often rewire their mindsets to perform better in their given sports and activities in order to transform themselves completely. To achieve the hardwiring, we must make the commitment to adhere to the following in the order of **imagination, visualization, practice,** and constant **repetition.** Our minds and bodies achieve what we desire when we constantly repeat what we want, when we start seeing the progress and start conquering what has been holding us back for so long. Again, this isn't difficult. It is as easy as *imagining* yourself in a near future moment, *visualizing* yourself with a body you're proud of, and *practicing* this technique over and over again (*repeating*). You will feel the positive motion and joy within your body as you imagine your best self. This is your body becoming excited about what is real in your imagination, and both your mind and body will want to move toward that great image of yourself. Repetition and habituation will transform your whole body.

The Role of Our Conscious Mind

After analyzing the subconscious mind, let us unpack the role of the conscious mind in our logical decision-making. Our conscious mind gives us what it thinks we want, what it thinks is best for us. The words we use matter when we talk to ourselves. Our mind is always attentive to the words we use. If we are using words of fear, doubt, and discouragement towards ourselves, we don't succeed. Our mind's job is to save us, to keep us alive. On the other hand, using empowering words towards ourselves will help us accomplish things we never thought possible.

Our conscious mind is focused on what we are currently aware of, the situation or obstacle at hand. So, let me use an example in the area of strength training and attempting to increase the maximum weight we lift in a gym. Once we allow doubt or fear into our mind, we will no longer be able to execute the routine before us due to the message of doubt the mind received. The moment doubt, fear, and discouragement enter us, we stop our progress, and the mind makes lifting the weight impossible. In a positive scenario, we would speak uplifting words: *I'm amazing, I am strong, I can lift this weight, I am confident, I can endure all things.* With words like this we have eliminated the "nonexistent" barrier of fear, doubt, and impossibility from the situation.

If we've failed at something in the past, why do we still carry the incident that occurred within us, as if it defines who we are? Why do we still latch on to these past fears and allow them to hinder us, making it hard to overcome them? The answer is that our brain is watching us and listening to us, and it wants to do anything in its power to try and help us reach our goal or keep us from executing something that might harm us. That is our mind acting based on logic and programs that were created in the subconscious mind over the years. The mind creates doubt as a protection mechanism in hopes to keep us safe (and even away from the pain of failure). At least that's what it is thinking.

At times our mind is trying to keep us safe from ourselves. It's always working on behalf of logic, whether good or bad, always trying to keep us happy, wanting what has always been familiar in our lives. Having said this, if our familiar is extra weight that we wish we didn't have, we need a shift in our mindset as our mind is striving to keep things within our familiar comfort zone, whether we like it or not.

Our Conscious Mind and Weight Loss

Our mind wants us to be comfortable in an array of areas, including weight loss. Weight issues might have been programmed into us due to foods being used either in celebrating an emotion or healing a disappointment. Often unwittingly, parents do this. If their kids perform well, they take them out to eat sugary, typically unhealthy meals because they create a sense of happiness. They are not bad parents, and they are often unaware that they are creating an addiction, a quick fix, stacking the happiness of an accomplishment with the happiness generated from consuming sugary food. With sugar as an indicator of celebration, our brains start releasing heightened amounts of endorphins, the brain's happy chemical. Food addiction may be one of the causes of obesity and related underlying conditions in both children and adults alike, creating all kinds of health problems related to high carb and sugary meals. It's a self-inflicted medical substitute to all kinds of feelings and emotions that we all deal with.

Unconsciously creating links between food and happiness is not new. Most children, teens, young adults, and adults have experienced this occurrence at some point. Not only can this habit become an addiction, thanks to all the celebrating of our minor accomplishments as we grow, other experiences begin to fall into this food reward system. Positive and/or negative experiences such as birthdays, promotions, awards, winning or losing in sports, passing or failing school, getting fired, falling in love and heartbreaks, investment flops, thriving and broken marriages, and losses due to unexpected tragic events also lead to food-related rewards. Then once again we find refuge in what makes us feel good during events where our family or friends gather with us. No one ever hears that someone's heart was broken, and they decided to eat ten heads of lettuce. Why? Because that was not what was presented to anyone as a feel-good celebration-type food during their developmental years.

So here we are now, possibly wanting to shed some pounds. If this is you, there is a solution. First, you need to start reprogramming your relationship with food and stop seeing food as a monster. Second, create small changes. Give yourself time with the new change, and once that becomes familiar to you, then make another small change. Third, continue this routine until you have managed to rewire your relationship with food. Not only are you going to look great, but you are going to feel so good that even the decisions you make will start matching the confidence, admiration, and love that you have created for yourself. And finally, stop using hurtful words towards yourself. Stop calling yourself fat and start saying you are on your path to health. The changes in words create changes in imagination, which completely changes your reality.

The Final Connection

Our mindset, emotions, and grit intertwined with our subconscious and conscious minds lead us to address our weight loss goals and other performance accomplishments. It really is easy. If we're not already in a positively pointed mindset, we need to shift our mindset. We need to uncover the why of any negative emotions that could be holding us back from embracing positivity. Seeing as weight loss and other performance accomplishments won't happen by themselves, this is where grit comes into play. It does take work to reach any positive result, but with grit and determination, this work seems easy as we desire to see the real-world outcomes that we can imagine in our minds.

Anything we want to change in our life to obtain the life that we desire for ourselves is possible. Keeping in mind that absolutely everything must come into play in our lives and work together to transform us into the unique individual that we want to be. We do have a say in our process. Whether it is learning how to use the full spectrum of how our mind works or performing better in life. It may be mental growth, working on achieving a health transformation via fitness and nutrition, or paying attention to the messages our body sends. With mindset, emotions, and grit, everything comes together so that we can obtain the successful healthy body we all want. A healthy body and mind will allow each of us to live a more fulfilled life. Remember, the past is gone, and the time to start is now!

About the Author

Jeannie Ruiz is a motivational speaker on food addiction (emotional eating and the effects of verbal abuse). She is also an L-1 CrossFit coach and is currently taking classes under Marisa Peer RTT (rapid transformational therapy) in hypnotherapy. During her spare time, she performs consultations on weight loss, focusing on low carb, keto, intermittent fasting, and carnivore diets, as well as healthy eating and lifestyles.

Jeannie's primary goal is to help others understand that they are beautifully and wonderfully made, that everyone deserves to find happiness, first in loving who they are and then finding happiness in their surroundings. She loves to work with people who are willing to take the next step in healing their bodies and transforming their lives.

Jeannie's message to everyone is that anyone can work to their full potential, but there is always more to gain. Our potential continues to strengthen and grow over time as we continue to dedicate ourselves to what we want in life, such as our goals, passions, dreams, and a healthier lifestyle and body. It does not matter where we begin but how we repeatedly work to enhance our situations that matters.

Email: itsjeannieruiz@gmail.com
Website: www.Itsjeannie.com
Instagram: https://www.instagram.com/jeannieruiz/

CHAPTER 24

DETOXIFICATION: MORE IMPORTANT THAN NUTRITION TODAY

By Christina Santini, CN, CTT, RYT
Clinical Nutritionist specializing in Biological Medicine
Copenhagen, Denmark / Los Angeles, CA

Everything in excess is opposed to nature.
—Hippocrates

We are living in a world where we are ever more obsessed with what we eat, yet ignorant of the toxins we're putting in our bodies.

Environmental Toxins Are Creating an Epidemic of Chronic Diseases

Chronic diseases have reached an epidemic high. Even though acute symptom handling is better than ever, cures of the root causes of many diseases today leave much to be desired. This is the most missed message in conventional and natural medicine today.

The Difference Between Treating Symptoms vs. Causes

If we want to be effective in treating diseases, we need to connect the dots back to the actual cause of the myriad of symptoms many of us have gotten used to accepting as part of being alive today—migraines, mood issues, digestive disorders, food "allergies," chronic pain, brain fog, sleep disturbances, fertility issues, weight-loss resistance, or weight-gain inability, etc.

The so-called chronic conditions people live with every day need not be chronic. They are only chronic because we are focused on treating the symptoms. Just as a car with a broken engine won't get better from top-quality gasoline, so too is our body: food and medicine alone are rarely enough.

The human body is often very capable of healing itself, unless it is blocked in some way. We don't need to eat fanatically to gain health. Food is medicine and can activate or inactivate genes of disease. Yet too many of us have gotten focused on the wrong priority of things in our quest for health. In many cases, we overcompensate in extremist diets without understanding the drivers of our health imbalances, and our relationship with food has gotten more toxic.

Today, more and more people eat fanatically than ever before. Cutting out entire food groups in the name of health, for example. Many of the current diet trends work only to promote binary thinking when it comes to food and our health—either we are vegan or carnivore, either we are high-fat or low-fat. And cutting out whatever food group is on trend is supposed to "save us." Yet these diet trends only seem to fade and repeat similar to other trends, for instance, fashion trends.

We may get some relief of symptoms by avoiding common allergens like dairy, wheat, and eggs, but anyone who starts eating more whole-food based ingredients will experience positive benefits regardless of which diet they choose. Eating easier-to-digest foods will make a difference for a compromised digestive system. However, it will not cure the cause, and the restrictive eating will become necessary if we want to keep symptoms at bay. Unless we treat the cause of our weak digestive system, nothing will really change.

How we react to a newfound diet trend will also depend on our own diet history. Our body biochemically adapts to how we eat to a certain extent. If we have been vegan for a long time and suddenly eat meat, our body may experience discomfort, simply because our digestive enzymes have changed over time. This is not proof that meat is bad, but proof that our body adapts to our diet, and this can lead us astray from what we actually need, i.e., more protein.

It is not uncommon to get client cases, where they have followed some extreme diet and tell a story about, how this has worked great for them, yet now "all of a sudden" their hormones are nonexistent and their hair is falling out (a typical low-fat vegan paradigm over time) or the typical long-term keto diet follower who tells a story about "sudden" weight-loss resistance, sleep issues, and often horrible triglyceride and cholesterol levels. Ironically the first couple of months on a keto diet result in much improvement in the same parameters. A keto diet does result in lower oxidative stress over the short term (less than six months), but long term it results in more oxidative stress (early aging, etc.). According to statements from 2016 to 2020 in the following three journals, *Nutrients, Cureus Journal of Medical Science,* and *Acta Neurologica Belgica*, levels of 4 HNE begin to accumulate over time, which can cause damage in the mitochondria. This matters because our mitochondria are the body's energy-providers, and anything that causes mitochondrial damage will cause a domino effect of health issues. They help repair damaged cells, detox and signals to our immune system to fight infection.

We have this polarized belief that either ONLY ketones are the body's true source of energy (proponents of keto diets) or ONLY glucose is the true source (high-carb diet proponents). Reasoning that "because something is good, more is better" can have negative or even fatal results.

The truth is, as shown in journals *Biochem* and *Nutrition*, too much of both glucose and ketones can be damaging. According to *Cardiology*, often the initial health effects we see on extreme diets are simply due to the fact people cut out processed foods and simple carbs and eat more whole food. What we keep forgetting is—what works in the short term doesn't necessarily work in the long run.

Eating with common sense and seasonally is now called carb cycling. Naturally, humans would cycle their carbs, fat, and protein throughout the seasons. Because too much of anything is a bad thing, as is too little of anything. Our own balance is found in feeding our body according to our current nutritional needs and goals. Long-term extremism when it comes to diets is never a good solution.

Your Personal Eating Analysis

I want you to think back to how you have been eating for the last ten years (because good or poor health doesn't happen overnight; it takes decades most often). I'm going to show you a tool I've used many times to help you identify where your food priorities should be focused. The tool is a SWOT (strengths, weaknesses, opportunities, and threats) health analysis of your current status that you complete in order to figure out what your next step should be.

In regards to your current health weaknesses, you will want to test this through a functional medicine provider if there are any "chronic symptoms," in order to not get stuck in symptom management. This is key to achieving a turnaround of your health in the long run.

The goal for change based on our analysis is to focus on small intentional steps that you are able to do consistently every day. Change doesn't happen overnight and you will fail if you don't accept this boring truth. Your next step to better health needs to be so easy that there are simply NO excuses to not do it. Don't be addicted to your bad habits and excuses; get your brain addicted to good habits, i.e., small consistent steps done every day to nourish and support you. That is the only way lasting change happens.

To identify what that next step looks like for you, let's do a SWOT analysis of your health.

Your SWOT Health Analysis

The first step in this exercise is to identify your health goal. Let's say your goal is to lose 20 pounds and become migraine-free. To reach this goal, you will now map out your strengths, weaknesses, opportunities, and threats as they relate to you reaching your health goal. Here is an example:

Strengths

- I live biking distance to work.
- I like vegetables if they are cooked in butter.
- I can do anything for 15 minutes daily.
- I can get the root causes of my issues "tested," so I know what I am doing makes sense.
- Instead of focusing on contradictory diets, I will focus on whole foods.

Weaknesses

- I have migraines.
- I have brain fog.

- I have weight-loss resistance.
- I have mold toxicity (test; don't guess), which affects both my weight and migraines.

Opportunities

- I will TEST to see what is causing the issue, so I can plan my small steps strategically (mold toxicity in this case).
- I will set aside 15 minutes to go for a walk every morning and evening.
- I will make sure I get up from sitting every hour to avoid metabolic dip by sitting for more than an hour in a row.
- I can pre-make a nightly whole-food-based sweet treat to cater to my cravings. e.g., a fruit salad with dark chocolate chunks + salted almonds. ALWAYS replace; don't just eliminate.

Threats

- I get depressed/lethargic during winter and can't follow through on much.
- I work long hours at a desk-job every day.
- I crave something sweet at night.
- I don't like to eat things that taste bad.
- I have failed over and over. I can't do it myself. I need accountability (coach, personal trainer, friend).

It is key for the SWOT analysis of your current health status to work so that you unravel the cause of your current health struggles. This may require testing, so you are sure you are taking baby steps in the right direction. Otherwise, your brain, which is pleasure-oriented, will look for quick fixes to procrastinate. If we are merely treating the symptoms—i.e., focusing on calorie-restriction over chemical disruption substances, which affect metabolism—regardless of that being through food, natural medicine, and/or conventional medicine, then we are putting in too much effort for not enough impact. And we get attached to our restrictive eating to avoid a symptom flare-up.

Maximum Impact with Minimum Effort

A healthy body can deal with a burger and fries. The question is: HOW do we achieve a healthy body that is in balance and is not sensitive to a million different foods and does not experience distress if we stray from our diet of choice? What I want to dig in to is getting maximum impact with minimum effort by addressing the root cause of our health or by preventing genetic disposition and helping genetic determination.

Our genes are NOT our destiny. We all have genes of diseases in us but not everyone gets sick from those diseases. This is largely due to the triggers we are exposed to throughout our life. This comes down to toxic load. Varied and whole-food-based nutrition, exercise, stress management, supplements, and "superfoods" all play a role in optimizing our health, but we need to start from the bottom up. A marathon runner doesn't start by running a marathon; they start by improving their 5K racing and in small increments, they build up their stamina to win. An Olympic weightlifter doesn't do their first ever clean-and-jerk with 200 pounds. They start with a 45-pound training bar and work their way up to their maximum weight. The exact same pattern holds true for everything else in life, including how we optimize our health.

Too many of us buy expensive supplements and focus on extreme diets instead of focusing on our core weakness, i.e., the domino piece that makes all the other pieces fall over. If you want to get the pieces to stand up, you don't start by focusing on a centerpiece, but the first piece that fell and affected a dozen other pieces (symptoms). We need to get better at logical reasoning because no amount of education can provide this for us, as we have seen time and time again in health care. We are trained in treating symptoms, pieces of the body isolated and away from the whole. This works somewhat for suppressing symptoms, but it leaves us addicted to whatever is suppressing our symptoms, until we have cured the cause.

According to *Alternative Medicine Review* and *The Journal of Integrative Medicine*, toxins are one of the biggest culprits of chronic disease. If we don't test for what is affecting our health, treatment becomes superficial. And, according to *Environmental Health Preview*, we are not testing for toxicity in most cases today. Practitioners often get lost in testing for trickle-down effects: mitochondrial dysfunction, gut damage, neurotransmitter imbalance, hormonal issues, inflammation markers, low thyroid. Yes, as shown in *BMC Pharmacology and Toxicology*, NONE of these answers the question WHY. Why are your hormones out of whack? Why are you suffering with low thyroid? Why is your gut flora aggressive? These are merely side effects of something else going on. And as long as we can ask WHY, we have not reached the cause of our health issue yet.

A proper cause analysis would go like this: I have digestive disorder. Why do I have this symptom? Because testing has revealed I have small intestinal bacterial overgrowth (SIBO). Why do I have SIBO? Testing for causative factors of aggressive gut flora has revealed I have mold toxicity. Why do I have mold toxicity? Mold toxicity stems from exposure to water-damaged buildings. Now we are at the source, and the source needs to be eliminated before treatment can begin. In this case, it would mean making sure you are not currently exposed to mold where you are living and/or working.

Environmental medicine deals with people exposed daily to small dosages of multiple compounds. In most cases, none of these levels are high enough to cause toxicity per se, but they still cause chronic health issues over time. The dose and exposure time is critical to determine whether something is toxic. Our biggest problem today being, we know very little about the synergy between all the different compounds, and also we don't understand what "safe levels" are over time. Many of these compounds might be things we are exposed to through decades of drinking contaminated water, living in water-damaged buildings, mercury from dental fillings, second-hand smoke inhalation, or eating meat contaminated with clostridia or glyphosate from non-organic grain. The top five sources of toxins linked to chronic disease today are:

1. Contaminated drinking water
2. Mold from living in a water-damaged building (mold can colonize your body even after you have moved out of suspect living condition)
3. Mercury dental fillings (the mercury is still in your body even if fillings are no longer there; removal needs to be done right to avoid a future toxicity issue)
4. Clostridia from conventional farming of pork and beef products (choose high-quality organic brands)
5. Non-organic grain products (source of glyphosate linked to digestive disorders, gluten being completely a secondary trigger if the gut already is damaged)

And then there is smoking or second-hand smoking. If you smoke, your biggest health change will be to stop smoking or to stop exposing yourself to second-hand smoke. Smoking completely inhibits the body's ability to detox by inactivating the MTHFR gene. This means no healthy eating makes up for any of the above toxic load culprits. And it is so much easier to detox your body from the compounds mentioned above than to accept a limiting life where your body is never fully functioning and where you are constantly required to eat a limited selection of foods to merely manage the symptoms. Yes, eating a bland diet void of grains, red meat, and dairy will be easier to digest, but it is NOT the only solution. Once your body is rid of blockages and your digestion functions, food does not have to be 100% clean. You can have your cinnamon roll and thrive, body, mind and soul too. But only when you figure out your weakest link and address it.

It is key that we identify our own core weakness and the causative factor for proper health care. Toxins can be eliminated when we know what we are treating. The current trend of "detoxing" without knowing what we are de-toxing from makes no sense. We won't detox just by following a 21-day juice fast. We need to know WHAT we are detoxing from and follow a matching strategy for that, in addition to testing before and after to ensure that what we are doing is working.

Here is a client example of chronic health issues due to toxicity. Through imaging before and approximately six months after treatment, we can see a snapshot of a client who came in with acute chemical toxicity. Chemicals typ-ically reach us through contaminated drinking water. This client was dealing with a host of systemic issues including a digestive disorder. Six months later, the testing showed her toxic values were in normal range and the symptoms reported were gone. Seemingly her "chronic" diagnosed issues were not so chronic when simply addressing the root cause. The client noted a difference the moment she added a water filter to her showerhead. She was bathing every day, year after year, in toxins that entered her bloodstream through her skin. Yet because these compounds often result in digestive distress, the focus was on restrictive diet patterns, which never cured the cause in the first place. It wasn't a dietary issue, it was an issue with toxic load.

In another example, a heavy metal test was done on a client with various psychiatric issues. This client was NOT crazy, but his brain toxicity was. Acute mercury and lead poisoning had gone undetected. Medication only offered little relief, and he did not benefit from therapy. We needed to treat the cause (in this case, heavy metal toxicity) rather than managing symptoms with medication and therapy. Again, in this situation, the symptom seemed like a psychiatric problem but was found to be another issue of toxicity.

As we can see, finding the real problem behind the symptoms is key. In this chapter, I've just touched the surface, but today we are surrounded by toxins. From the obvious things like polluted water, polluted air, mold, asbestos, and lead to less known toxins in cleaning and even beauty products. If you suffer from something, but you don't know exactly what it is, don't accept the "chronic" symptoms you're living with. Begin your search for the root cause of your ailment. Once identified, start moving toward your successful body by performing the health SWOT analysis. By knowing what it is you are targeting, you can implement small daily steps to remove the blockages limiting your potential for optimal health. When you move the focus from symptom to cause, your body and mind moves away from narrow-minded thinking and acting. Instead of being in this dark world focusing only on eating disorders and restrictive diets, you can create a life where you enjoy food and reach toxic-free optimal health and well-being.

About the Author

Christina Santini is owner of The Nutrition Clinic with an office in Copenhagen and a pop-up office in Los Angeles, California. She has a degree in human nutrition from Metropolitan University College, Copenhagen and was certified in biological medicine from Paracelsus Academy by Dr. Rau in Switzerland and in medical thermography and yoga in California.

Christina has been one of the first practitioners in Europe to test for environmental toxins. She has worked at private hospitals in Europe, New York, and Los Angeles. She does workshops for patient organizations, writes articles in various outlets, and speaks at conferences internationally. Clients have included Forbes 500 and "Wall Street Wolves," and she's also been the last stop for sufferers of "chronic" diseases. Christina Santini is passionate about the science-based overlapping between Western medicine and Eastern health philosophy. She splits her time between Copenhagen and Los Angeles with her fiancé, Peter, and cat, Spencer.

Email: info@ChristinaSantini.com
Website: www.ChristinaSantini.com

CHAPTER 25
SAVED BY THE BELL

By Paul Scianna, CPT
Owner of Empowering Punch Fitness, Professional Boxer
Strongsville, Ohio

*Life's not about how hard of a hit you can give ... it's about
how many you can take, and still keep moving forward.*
—Sylvester Stallone

One, one-two, one-two-three, drop-two-three, one-slip, two-three-four-five. To most, those are just random sequences of numbers blurted out without rhyme or reason. To my clients, however, those numbers represent a battle call in the war against weight.

I have been in love with the sport of boxing for as long as I can remember. My grandfather put a pair of gloves on me when I was 3, and immediately, I felt invincible. Ironically, as I was always small for my age, I often got picked on due to my stature. Dealing with that inferiority complex, my insecurities skyrocketed, and school became a constant struggle. Always feeling behind or judged, my anxiety and lack of focus continued to get the best of me. I was far from invincible.

Now, at the gym ... that's a different story. The boxing gym was my sanctuary, my confidence, my invincibility. Boxing is you against you. And you, and only you, can seal the fate of what happens when that bell rings. How hard are you going to hit the bag today? How fast and how strong? Who or what are you going to let into your mind to affect the outcome? That is what I love the most about boxing. Most people cannot comprehend their true potential until they are forced to dig deep into the depths of their being to fight for what they want.

Boxing has an invaluable "Miyagi" effect in that it subconsciously strengthens from the inside out. Yes, we use it for sport and exercise, but the results my clients have attained from boxing workouts far surpass the aesthetics.

Where There's a Will, There's a Way.

My first client when I moved to Cleveland was a woman named Vicky. Vicky was 29 and had been trying to pass the physical ability test to get into the police academy. She was coming up short on some of the fitness scores, but her main concern was her weight. She needed to lose 19 pounds to pass the weight requirement for the test, which was in seven days. Being a boxer, cutting weight was a common theme for me, but typically you have time to prepare and plan a training regime; we, unfortunately, did not have that luxury. I told Vicky it could be done, but it was going to be grueling and exhausting. I also had to factor in that she had to perform well in the physical test at the end of the week, so I needed to make sure she wasn't over-trained and too weak to compete.

Vicky's preparation for her test was a case of mind over matter. We trained two to three times per day, ensuring she had ample rest time in between sessions and was well nourished to properly recover. We boxed every night for six days in a row. With every punch, she got stronger and stronger, but it wasn't physical, it was all mental. We both knew six days was not enough time to build physical strength, so her training turned into a mental feat. I watched the determination in her eyes as she hit my mitts, punch after punch. The crack of the gloves fueled the fire inside her and allowed her body to keep pushing.

She did it. She not only lost 19 pounds in 6.5 days, she passed all her physical requirements beating her previous scores. She is still a proud member of the Cleveland Police Department today.

Size Doesn't Matter

If I'm known for anything, it is my direct approach. Being a competitive athlete, you are always given the raw truth, even when it hurts. I'm often ridiculed for taking this approach with my clients, as I never sugarcoat the facts. To me, that only prolongs the problem and hinders the solution. If you have been battling weight your entire life and everyone keeps telling you it's okay, you will begin to think it's okay. Well, it's not okay. It's *not* okay because it's dangerous and unhealthy, and I'm *not* okay with allowing anyone to settle for being unhealthy and unsafe.

Terence was a 429-pound man that came to my gym day after day. He was this pleasant, jovial human being with a beaming personality. He didn't exhibit the typical insecurities that usually accompany someone of his size. Usually, I would commend someone for having such a positive attitude and level of self-confidence; however, in this case, it was a dangerous detriment. Terence had a good job, was happily married, and led a seemingly fulfilling life. The only problem was that he was a ticking time bomb from a health perspective.

After months of watching his unsuccessful efforts of coming to the gym and going through the motions, I pulled him into my office and said very candidly, "If you don't do something about your weight now, you're going to die." I know now I took a gamble with the blunt delivery, but I knew his strong personality and figured I had to hit him straight if I had any chance of helping.

Thankfully, Terence had also been watching me for months and knew my words were only coming out of concern. He just looked at me and said, "Okay." He was in. He respected the fact that I was the only one who didn't avoid the obvious. I made a deal with him; I told him if he did everything I told him, I promised he would lose 200 pounds in one year. I don't think he fully believed me, but out of respect for me and my efforts to help him, he agreed.

Due to his size, his options for exercises were limited. He couldn't get on the floor because he couldn't get back up. He couldn't fit on many of the machines in the gym, and he had weak knees from carrying around such excess weight for so many years. It almost seemed impossible, but it wasn't.

So, we boxed! One, one-two, one-two-three, two-three, two-three, slip-five. These are boxing combinations. One is your left jab, two is your right hand, three is your left hook, four and five are uppercuts. Boxing has no size limit; it's just you and the bag. You can punch as light or as hard as you can, you can speed up, slow down, and take a break when needed.

Boxing works every muscle group in your body. It keeps your heart racing, improves your focus and coordination, and builds strength and endurance. Terence couldn't run around the track, but he could hold his own in my boxing class with 20 other members who were half his size. Boxing creates an even playing field and never discriminates.

Terence lost his first 100 pounds in five months. He was on a mission. As exciting of a journey it had been up until that point, it began to get rocky. As the pounds were fading away, his emotions were surfacing. The real reasons why he had allowed himself to become that size and the fear of failure, of falling back into old habits and lifestyles, were becoming alarmingly apparent. The first phase was mostly physical and just following the fitness and nutrition plans. Eventually, he was battling the mental and emotional aspects that reveal themselves with the process. Some of our most productive sessions were just talking and really flushing out how and why his weight overcame his life for so long.

Terence did hit his goal of losing 200 pounds that year, but the true accomplishment was not on the scale. He was a wrestling enthusiast when he was younger but never had a chance to compete due to his size. That same year, at age 45, he enrolled in Baldwin Wallace College and walked onto their wrestling team as their starting heavyweight wrestler.

Class Clown

One of the most disheartening characteristics for me with my weight loss clients is what I call "class clown." That's when it's easier to just make fun of yourself because of your size, rather than do something about it. My client, Allyson, always called herself the "funny fat girl," which killed me because she hid behind that reputation. She was beautiful inside and out, had many friends, a very loving family, and was the life of the party. But, despite her efforts to present herself as happy and content with her life, she was miserable. She was too embarrassed to go to a gym, so I trained her in her living room.

Also, due to her weight and bad knees, she was extremely limited in her movements. She started with me at 350 pounds and was extremely deconditioned. Being overweight most of her life, she struggled with even envisioning herself at a healthy range. She was very skeptical and frustrated with herself because she had so many limitations.

Allyson's results started slowly because she wasn't fully committing to her routine. Once she hit a couple milestones—20 pounds, 40 pounds, etc.—her weight wasn't so funny anymore. The more she boxed, the more she began to let go of the pent-up anger she had towards herself for allowing it to go on for so long. Allyson, being the "funny fat girl" (her words), was always the third wheel at social events since she never had a boyfriend.

Allyson's goal, although it took her awhile to admit it, was to feel confident enough with her body to actually start dating. She had been ashamed of the way she looked for so long that she was terrified to get into a serious relationship, and she did not have the self-esteem to even attempt any interactions. After about 15 months, she had lost 160 pounds and was beaming. My wife even took her shopping to buy new clothes for her first date. She is currently happily married and just had her first child.

Non-Scale Victories

When we talk about non-scale victories, my client Dick gets the gold star. He had been a member at the gym where I worked for years and had some heart health issues. He shared with me that he had a blocked artery and was determined to avoid surgery by improving his fitness and nutrition.

Dick was 70 years old when he started training with me. He boxed, weight-trained, and we managed his diet to ensure he wouldn't need to go under the knife. He did his first ever pullup at the age of 76. Dick continued to work with me until he was 84 years old when he moved out of state.

Dick never had the surgery and never had an issue again, rather he took control over the success of his own body. His doctor told him, "Whatever you're doing, keep doing it!" Dick just chuckled under his breath not knowing if he should reveal to his doctor that he was boxing. Dick was victorious, indeed.

Five More Years

Marie was a long-time client and a picture of health. She followed my program flawlessly, as she loved the way she felt when she was in shape and strong. One day, I received a panicked call from her with the news that she had been diagnosed with stage 4 colon cancer. Her doctors told her she had a couple months to live because it was so advanced when they caught it. Marie was in shock, to say the least. "How did this happen to me?" she kept crying to me, and with good reason.

Marie did everything right … ate right, exercised, led a healthy lifestyle … Some things just can't be explained. I was at a loss for words, as I too, was in shock from the news. All I could think to tell her was to fight. Statistics are just that, statistics. The mind is an immensely powerful tool, and when all the odds are against you, you dig deep, and you *fight*.

She began her chemo treatments, which, of course, made her terribly ill and weak. It was unbearable seeing her so weak and frail, as she was always a wall of lean muscle and energy, but we knew it would get worse before it got better. And it did. She kept her spirit up and kept telling me to save her a spot in class.

After a few months of treatment, she began to show signs of improvement. The cancer stopped spreading, and she even went into remission. Our whole gym was familiar with her story, so the first time she stepped back into the boxing ring, there was a roar of applause combined with tears of joy from most. The doctor once told her that the only reason she has been able to fight with the strength she did was due to her health coming into the battle. Marie lived five beautiful years longer than they predicted upon her grave diagnosis.

Agoraphobia

Gene called my gym one day asking about boxing classes. He explained he had agoraphobia and was very anxious in crowds but was determined to learn how to box. We suggested one of our lower-attended classes that moved at a slower pace, figuring it would allow him more time to acclimate. He was clearly uneasy but continued to fight through his urges to retreat, as he was fascinated with the teachings.

Fast-forward six years and several hundred classes later, Gene just passed his personal training certification course and also applied for a position with us, so he can share his experience and pass along what he's learned. He, to this day, claims that boxing is what cured him of his disorder.

Fit Kids Box

We have several success stories pertaining to children, which I will keep anonymous to protect their privacy; however, the results are important to note. We've had several children with autism that have flourished because of the focus and the learned ability to go at their own pace and the intense outlet for energy release that boxing provides. I've counseled many parents of children with eating disorders, teaching them how to incorporate fitness and nutrition into their kids' lives.

Boxing is fun for kids. They get a tremendous workout, and they don't even realize they're exercising. And our most popular youth participants are those getting bullied. I was there. I know the signs ... the acting out, the shame, the fear, and embarrassment that can traumatize young minds and souls forever. We teach how to fight back … only physically when *absolutely* necessary, but more so by building their confidence and self-esteem, so they are no longer targets. We teach them a skill they can be proud of and so they can feel safe knowing they are in control of their bodies and they are no longer victims.

I could go on and on with hundreds of examples of how fitness, nutrition, and having the right coach in your corner can provide so much more than a smaller waistline and some nice biceps. We all want to look good on the outside, but if that strength and shine isn't reciprocated on the inside, you have a *dangerous* imbalance. I was taught at an early age that if you want something badly enough, you *fight* for it. My job is to teach those who want to live a healthy, confident, and fulfilling lifestyle how to fight to get it, and the rewards of seeing people fight and get the health and confidence they are after is priceless.

About the Author

Paul Scianna is the owner of Empowering Punch Personal Training and Fitness Studio where he developed his own unique recipe to transform both mindset and the body in a manner conducive for all ages, sizes, and fitness levels. He's responsible for literally thousands of pounds of weight loss from his extensive list of transformed clients.

With his debut as a professional boxer on the reality TV show, *The Next Great Champ*, with Oscar De La Hoya, Paul's true area of expertise lies within his teaching style. He breaks down the science in layman's terms to ensure every client not only understands how to follow the process, but more importantly, learns from it. His unmatched work ethic and perseverance to succeed is the reason he is so highly sought out in the world of fitness. His programs empower you with the knowledge, confidence, and desire to never give up on yourself again.

For anyone wanting to experience Paul's Empowering Punch, go to https:// bit.ly/2IoBadh and enter the promo code **SUCCESS** for a complimentary month of live, virtual fitness classes.

Email: Paul@empoweringpunch.com
Website: www.empoweringpunch.com

CHAPTER 26
PERPETUAL MOTION

By Rocky Snyder, CSCS
Master Trainer, Author of *Fit to Surf* and *Return to Center*
Santa Cruz, California

We are what we repeatedly do. Excellence is not an act, but a habit.
—Aristotle

Step back for a minute and look at why we, as a society, are encouraged to exercise. I guess you could begin at any time in our history, but let's choose the Industrial Revolution as our starting point. Up until that time, most Americans were living in rural areas performing manual labor on farms and ranches. The average amount of physical activity could be easily measured in hours or an entire day. As decades passed and technology developed, more Americans moved away from the farm to make it big in the cities. Instead of toiling behind the plow blade, they stood for hours behind machines, pulling levers and turning wheels. Physical activity had reduced significantly to only a few hours a day.

Eventually, the assembly line began to become automated, and many Americans transitioned themselves into sitting for countless hours behind a desk. Physical activity had reached an all-time low as obesity, joint pain, tendinitis, and other maladies began to increase. Today's world is even more technologically advanced with countless ways to move less. People now measure their activity level in minutes or even seconds! Programs such as "8 Minute Abs," "Tabata Protocol," "4 Minutes to Fitness" are prime examples that even a handful of minutes may prove to be a challenge for most de-conditioned workers.

With this exponential diminishment of movement comes the breakdown of the human form. Most of the illnesses, aches, and pains in today's culture can be directly related to a lack of purposeful movement. Our society has reached such a point with its lack of movement that facilities were created to encourage movement back into a person's life: gyms.

So, we are told to go to a health club and get some exercise. After years of minimal physical activity, we become members of an exclusive spa. The entry level instructor gives you your "first workout" as part of your membership. Ironically, the workout involves pushing handles or elbow pads, pulling bars, lifting leg rollers, and pressing a metal plate with your feet—all while sitting on a comfortable, upholstered seat. I thought the problem was we were sitting too much? So, we go to a place to get exercise, and they have us sit? While there can be some great benefits in gym workouts, be wary of limiting yourself to repeated two-dimensional exercises while seated.

Most bodies do not need to experience more sitting. What most bodies need is to move with the least amount of restriction and the most amount of control in three-dimensional space. After months or years of living in this technologically advanced world, the human structure begins to get contorted away from its optimal position. We begin to see postural distortions that often lead to joint or soft tissue pain. If the situation is left unchecked, a person may elect to get surgical intervention to replace worn parts because of compromised movements.

Movement is the key to restoring function to the body and getting out of pain (not managing it). It does not necessarily mean you have to lift weights. In fact, some bodies are not in a state where weightlifting would be advantageous; it could be detrimental. What is important is to find educated professionals who are trained to restore proper movement back into the body.

Workout Considerations

Imagine sitting in a rowboat with two people. The two people are a small child and an NFL athlete. They are sitting beside each other, and both are pulling on their own oar. They are in perfect synchronicity. Their form is identical, yet the boat keeps traveling in circles. After a month of paddling, both rowers have grown stronger, but the boat keeps making circles. Obviously, the NFL athlete can generate more force than the child, and, unless the child grows in strength, comparable to the footballer, the boat will continue to circle.

What if, instead, we were discussing the strength differences in a person's arms rather than two different-sized rowers? Can you see the same outcome occurring? We need to be mindful of this as most people have a dominant arm and leg. If, like almost everyone in this country, you have subtle imbalances and distortions in your resting posture, and your gym routine is only comprised of bilateral exercises, expect to reinforce muscular imbalances, postural distortions, compensatory movements, and structural weakening. The likelihood of sustaining an injury is just a matter of time.

The solution is to be mindful of your exercise routines. There should be a good reason for performing each exercise in your workout. You just need to ask why it is you are performing it. You may want to consider incorporating exercises that help to balance the body more. Perform single arm or leg exercises. Perhaps focus a little more attention on the weaker side. Try and move the arms in an alternating fashion or in opposing directions. Vary your movements often. These are simple suggestions which may provide long-term insurance against the side effects of bilateral movements.

The Goldilocks Place

Movement is an amazing thing we are all capable of doing. Watch any "People Are Awesome" video on YouTube, and you will be stunned at what the human form is able to do. Or watch any high-level athlete perform and notice how easy they make everything appear. When the body is highly conditioned and balanced, it is easier to perform complex actions. When joints are in their proper place, movement is almost effortless.

But what is a joint? What is an elbow or a knee, really? Have you ever stopped to think about it? Simply put, a joint is the space between bones. Sure, there are several types of soft tissue that surround the space—tendons, cartilage, ligaments, etc.—but ultimately it is the space itself and the shape of the bone surface which defines the joint. If there is too little space, there will be compression, wearing, and tearing. If there is too much space, there will be laxity, instability, and possibly dislocation. Which joint is healthier? The answer is neither. A joint with too much space is at just as much risk of injury as the joint with too little. So, there is this "Goldilocks" place in which all joints should ideally exist. It shouldn't be too little or too much, but just right.

The really interesting thing is how the subconscious part of the brain that regulates movement and structure will always strive for perfection. If the joints of the body have just the right amount of space, the brain will try and keep it that way. However, if the body suffers an injury, surgery, or is confined to one position for prolonged periods of time, the space of some joints may very well change. No matter what, the brain will find the best way to get around the issue in that moment.

It is not uncommon for someone with tight, compressed hips to have lower back or knee pain. If the hips are not able to move freely, then a neighboring joint like the back or knee may very well attempt to move more. Unfortunately, knees and lower backs are not meant to perform the work of the hips, hence, the painful reaction. Perhaps your neck is restricted rotating left to right, but greatly flexes side to side? One movement increases when another decreases, so it is important to strive to become aware of the restrictions in your body and work toward more healthy alignment. You might be shocked about how great you can feel by simply getting your body into correct alignment.

A Word About Movement

Riddle of the day: what does a river, a newspaper, and the human body all have in common?

Answer: things go bad when their circulation drops.

If water were to stop flowing down a river, it would eventually dry up and no longer exist. If nobody subscribed to a newspaper, the company would end up going out of business. Similarly, when the human body reduces circulation, a whole myriad of problems can ensue. These are the problems you often hear people, or find yourself, complaining about: joint pain, excessive muscle tension, tendinitis, restless legs, arthritis, low energy, shortness of breath, dizziness, neuropathy, numbness, and tingling.

There is a very simple remedy for many of these issues: it's called movement. In some cases, it might need to be a specific movement, but for most people, a simple walk can achieve wonders. Walking is what drives organic function. When we walk, all of the 206 bones, 360 joints, and over 650 muscles move through the full range of motion in three-dimensional space. The muscles create a pumping mechanism that helps circulate fluids (not just blood) throughout the body. It causes a greater uptake of oxygen and improves the overall gas exchange in our respiratory system. It can also help achieve better hormonal balance, digestion, and state of mind.

Try this little experiment some time when you have been inactive, like sitting at a desk for more than 30 minutes. Before getting out of the chair, perform a mental check-in with how your body feels. Are there any areas that ache or feel too much tension? What is your emotional state? How is your energy level? Are you alert, or is your mind tending to wander?

Now get up from the chair and go outside for a five-minute brisk walk. Maintain a gentle awareness of your surroundings and if your body experiences any kind of change. After five minutes, head back inside to your chair, but do not sit down. Stand by your chair and perform another mental check-in. Has anything changed? Are there more or less aches? How much tension are you experiencing? What is your emotional state? How is your energy level? Are you more or less alert?

If you noticed a change in any of these areas, you have proven the point. The body needs to move on a very regular basis. For most people, it needs to move more than it currently does. The cool thing about this little experiment is that it creates a noticeable change in a very short amount of time. The sad part is that the body will also revert back to its previous state if you sit back down for a long time. The key is to break up your time spent being inactive with short bursts of gentle activity. It will not only improve your circulation, but it will also improve your feeling of happiness.

Everything in Moderation

All too often I get asked the same question: "How many times a week should I exercise?" My answer is always the same, "Only those days which end in the letter Y." The person usually smiles and then asks, "What's the least amount of time per day I should exercise?" Never mind that the premise of their question is to find the smallest amount of effort required to lose weight or gain strength. They have been given the amazing gift of life in a body that can move, and they want to know the minimal amount to do. My answer to this second question also never changes, "Just for five minutes."

The person typically looks at me in amazement. They cannot believe that just five minutes a day is all they need to do. It's not all they need to do, but it's a start and more than they are presently doing. If I had told them that they needed to exercise one hour a day for five to six days per week, the chance of them adding this program to their already busy lifestyle would be impossible. However, if someone were to feel that the task is achievable with only five minutes a day, the likelihood of compliance is much greater.

My son has been taking guitar lessons for several years. Instead of telling him he needed to practice the guitar for 20 minutes and do the homework his teacher gave him, I just ask him to play me a song and see if I can guess what it is. It's just one song. It would take him maybe three minutes to play it. He ends up playing several renditions of "Name That Tune." Those three minutes turn into 15 to 20 minutes when he does not feel like it is a daunting task.

The same can be said of almost anything in our life. My grandfather used to paint one side of his house every year. That way every four years his house was completely repainted. Do you feel like reading *War and Peace*? Go ahead. Just read two pages a day. It may take you 613 days to finish it, but you'll be able to check that book off your bucket list eventually. Go for a five-minute walk and see how your body feels. You can keep going if you like it or not. At least you reached a doable goal.

People hope to achieve big goals without laying out the small steps that will get them there. Breaking down your goal into very small attainable steps might be a better approach. Nothing says you have to stop at one step either. Go ahead and perform the next step if you feel like it. The hard part comes when you make the steps too big to reach. What follows is a misstep, and you end up face down and feeling like you can't keep going. Just start with the first five minutes.

Goals and Giving Back

In 2017, my wife asked me what I would like to do for my 50th birthday. I told her the last thing I wanted was a party. Instead, I wanted to scratch something off my bucket list. I wanted to do something to keep my body moving. How about paddling 28.5 miles across deep water canyons in the Alaskan current, through great white shark- and orca-infested 54-degree water using only your arms as propulsion? I would set out from Santa Cruz Harbor on a journey across Monterey Bay in hopes of arriving on the other side at Del Monte Beach and Fisherman's Wharf. She said the insurance policy was paid up, so have at it. I shared the idea with a couple of like-minded, idiotic friends, and they surprised me by saying they would do it with me. I knew that the instant the words left my lips, I had to follow through with it.

Accomplishing goals with friends is ten times easier than doing it alone. We began paddle training earlier in the year through stormy winter conditions but eventually began to feel stronger and more confident. When it was suggested that we turn it into a fundraising event, there was no time needed to decide; of course, we would. Getting outside of myself, working with others for a common goal, and supporting a fantastic cause at the same time—where do I sign up? The Living Breath Foundation was founded by family members of some of my clients and the work they continue to do to help those with cystic fibrosis warrants as much support as possible.

By June of 2017, I had paddled countless miles in all sorts of conditions, and about 100 days remained until the group attempted the crossing. To be honest, there were moments when I just didn't want to keep going. Stiffness, aches, and pains that would not be there if I'd just kept my mouth shut. Dark, early mornings when I would rather stay in bed next to my wife than get up and jump in the 54-degree water for several hours. There were moments when I would rather surf with friends than go out and accumulate more miles.

Fortunately, moments pass and so too do the thoughts that try and defeat us. That tells us we can't do something. That nobody is going to care if we just stop. That it is okay if we just stay in bed this one morning instead of going out to paddle. If I listened to that inner voice of defeatism, it would be followed by regret and the question, "What if … ?" The secret is to let those thoughts roll on by, to not hold on to them. To keep doing what you are doing. They are sure to return, but if we keep letting them roll on by, we develop a pattern of success.

This pattern is contagious to other aspects of our life. Think of the people whom you view as successful. They could be men and women in sports, business, family life, or finance. Do they give up when faced with adversity, or do they find a way to keep going forward? How often do you think that Bill Gates, Steve Jobs, Michael Jordan, or Warren Buffett listened to that negative inner voice?

Yet how many people do you know who succumb to these negative, defeating thoughts and struggle with countless attempts to achieve what they want? These are people who make the same common mistakes:

- They attempt to do it by themselves.
- They lose focus on the goal.

- They do not break down the road to success into smaller, achievable steps.
- They place themselves low on the priority list.
- They believe everything they think.

Don't make these mistakes! No matter what your goal is, you can achieve it if you avoid these pitfalls. Have a support group and use it to its fullest. Keep your eyes on the prize. Break down each step into smaller steps, and if they seem too big, then break them down even more. Re-prioritize yourself and place that person at the top of the list. If you don't, everything will find a way to sneak up past you. Finally, don't believe everything you think. Ask a friend for advice and share your thoughts with a confidante. Jack LaLanne was once asked if he ever got tired of getting up every morning to exercise. His answer was, to paraphrase, "Hell yes! But I know if I don't the consequences are severe."

On September 29, 2017, we achieved our goal. Over 7.5 hours of constant paddling in 57-degree Alaskan current. Yes, our arms ached, and several people became hypothermic. five paddlers were sick, one with bronchitis and another with a 102-degree temperature. Yes, feet fell asleep and stinging tentacles amassed on our forearms. Yes, the conditions turned sour sooner than we preferred. Yet, we kept on going because one thought kept returning to everyone's mind: no matter what adversity we faced, it was nothing compared to what a person with cystic fibrosis has to endure daily. We dedicated ourselves to training our bodies, and we paddled across the bay because we could. We paddled for those who could not, not for ourselves. That is some of the best motivation going. If it is true that you can judge the person you are by the people with whom you surround yourself, then I am a very blessed and grateful person, and I live the life I love.

Now I challenge you to break the pattern of modern-day stillness, get your body in alignment, and move. You don't have to transform overnight. Set your goals, get someone to keep you accountable, and remember that even five minutes of walking is better than nothing. Build your own patterns of success and enjoy your life.

About the Author

Rocky Snyder is a certified strength and conditioning specialist. He is a nationally recognized expert in human movement with nearly 30 years of professional experience. Rocky has trained thousands of clients ranging from grandparents to professional athletes and Olympic champions. Aside from owning and operating his training studio in Santa Cruz, California, Rocky is the author of *Return to Center* and fitness books: *Fit to Surf, Fit to Paddle*, and *Fit to Ski & Snowboard*. Rocky continues to travel far and wide providing educational workshops to personal trainers, manual therapists, chiropractors, and physical therapists.

Email: rocky@rockysfitnesscenter.com
Website: www.rockysfitnesscenter.com

CHAPTER 27

THE PHYSIOLOGY OF RESISTANCE TRAINING

By Johnny Spilotro, CPT
Rehabilitation Specialist, Functional Fitness Coach
Las Vegas, Nevada

The harder I push, the more I find within myself. I am always looking for the next step, a different world to go into, areas where I have not been before.
—Ayrton Senna

Exercise in the world we inhabit today has become a most dire need. Due to sedentary lifestyles fueled by a high abundance of technology that supports a lack of movement, humans are facing serious health challenges. According to the researcher Fryar and his team, as reported in an article in *Preventative Medicine*, heart disease remains the leading cause of death in the United States. The article goes on to state that cardiovascular disease risk factors, such as high blood pressure, high cholesterol, diabetes, being overweight, obesity, can lead to fatal consequences. Metrics like this alone have persuaded many people to exercise vigorously, but the vast majority of people who exercise concentrate on fitness for weight loss. Most fall short of their goals. Whether it be weight loss or increased cardiorespiratory stamina, most people who exercise fail in reaching their goals due to the approach they take in their training methods. They believe in the old school of thought, which constitutes that cardio exercises are the best way to burn calories and lose fat mass. However, the latest research has shown that there is one effective method for burning fat that, in turn, improves an individual's overall fitness level: resistance training.

Resistance training is defined as an exercise modality that utilizes a form of weight working against the plane of gravity to elicit a muscular response. Not only has this method of training grown in popularity, researchers Kraemer and Ratamess found that resistance training is recommended by prominent national health organizations including the American College of Sports Medicine and the American Heart Association for most populations, from adolescents to the elderly, including those with cardiovascular or neuromuscular disease. The reason for such support for resistance training is that the general individual interested in it typically aspires for a body type or body performance like that of a professional athlete or a bodybuilder. With this kind of high aspiration, the individual can better stay engaged in their strength training regimen.

While resistance training may seem simple (because it is), each individual has their own limitations that need to be addressed when it comes to designing an effective exercise program that fits their needs and biological limitations. These include, but are not limited to, hormonal responses, metabolic rates, and caloric expenditure. Therefore, as stated in Kraemer and Ratamess's article in *Medicine and Science in Sports and Exercise*: "It is the magnitude of the individual effort and systematic structuring of the training stimulus that ultimately determines the outcomes associated with resistance training." In today's world, resistance training is boiled down to a science, both inside the body and out, and every factor is in consideration to effectively develop the ideal training program for the individual. Let's look into this more.

Geeking Out on Muscles

Like all the other major body systems, the nervous system goes hand in hand with the muscular system. The brain and spinal cord utilize countless branches of nerve endings to innervate all 640 skeletal muscles that help us stand erect, walk, reach and grab, produce heat, and protect our organs. To accomplish these functions, our muscles react to an external stimulus, regardless if it is simple, complex, planned, autonomous, at rest, or even during exercise. This stimulus is processed as an electrical impulse in our neurons. This is known as an action potential. In approximately five milliseconds, a single neuron can fire one of these action potentials via intercellular branches called dendrites and pass that sensory information to the threshold between a nerve ending and muscle tissue, called a neuromuscular junction, or in a smaller scale, a motor unit. So, when we exercise with resistance training, we're exercising a lot more than just the muscles. We're exercising the relationship between our brain, nervous system, and muscles simultaneously.

Sodium and potassium are two of the key minerals that apply to muscular function. Normally, positively charged potassium ions and negatively charged sodium ions are floating outside and inside the cell membrane, respectively. When the action potential crosses the threshold to a neighboring cell membrane, those ions switch positions through what is called a sodium-potassium pump, thus switching the charges of the cell. Once the action potential is finished, those cells transition back to their respective areas via diffusion. That moment when ions depolarize and repolarize occurs with every muscular contraction inside our bodies, regardless of rest or active states. There is a lot more going on than we normally think with even the smallest flexing of any muscle.

Muscle Contractions

There are three kinds of contractions that can occur in skeletal muscle that elicit strength and/or flexibility. There is the concentric contraction, which is a muscle shortening; the eccentric contraction, which is a muscle lengthening; and an isometric contraction, where the muscle is not changing length. These contractions occur in relation to what kind of joint they innervate, the direction the muscle fibers travel, and their primary function. For example, a bicep curl occurs when the biceps brachii pulls the resistance towards a decreasing joint angle in the elbow joint. However, to aid in extension the biceps lengthen their fibers to assist the increase in that particular joint angle. The muscle can also isometrically contract by simply holding the resistance for a long period of time without changing length.

All three of these contractions have varying effects on how a muscle behaves in terms of hypertrophy, or growing in size, elasticity, or tensile strength. As shown in the 2020 article "Recent Advances In Understanding Resistance Exercise Training—Induces Skeletal Muscle Hypertrophy in Humans," by researcher Joanisse and team, during the act of resistance training, "exogenous factors include RE-related variables (load, reps, time under tension, volume, etc.), diet-related variables such as protein supplementation, energy intake, and consumption of anabolic supplements (i.e., creatine)." This gives us an understanding of how nutrition and resistance training go hand in hand, an issue we look into in the upcoming section.

Fuel for Muscles

For an athlete who practices resistance training on a regular basis, carbohydrates are essential for giving the body energy not only for the muscles to operate, but for the brain to process information as well. Caloric needs are dependent on an individual's activities, but a person must keep in mind the kind of carbohydrates to ingest. Simple carbohydrates are similar to small bamboo shacks in that they are much easier for the elements (or in this case, the body's metabolism) to break down. In contrast, complex carbohydrates are similar to skyscrapers such as the Empire State Building, due to the fact that they are composed of larger molecular structures that will require more time and effort for metabolic processes to catabolize them (or break them down, in the case of skyscrapers). Sugars stemming from foods such as rice, sweet potatoes, greens, and fruits are converted into an energy source called adenosine triphosphate (ATP) that is used up by the muscles by generating heat. This unit of heat is quantified as a familiar term called "calories."

During strenuous exercise, muscle fibers will inflict small microscopic tears that elicit a small soreness occurring roughly 24 to 48 hours after the exercise session. This phenomenon is called delayed onset muscle soreness (DOMS). To combat DOMs and to help expedite the recovery process, protein sources such as red meat, chicken, fish, beans, and other forms of poultry, are metabolized in the muscles in an effort to rebuild the previously "injured" muscles from the workout.

Muscle soreness is only one of the determinants that defines improvements in muscular strength and efficiency since as the micro-tears in muscle are repaired, the repairing materials are what adds size to the muscle, a desired outcome of many resistance training practitioners. A major key factor in strength training is the periodization, or planning, of a training program for a person's specific goals. Strength, hypertrophy (increase in muscle fiber size), weight loss, and flexibility all require different schematics when it comes to coaches and trainers planning exercise programs for their athletes.

Building Muscle Size

Hypertrophy, or the enlargement of muscles, is a popular goal for the general population, as most people desire to have more definition in respective areas, especially for men, in the arms and chest. There is no set range that clearly defines the ideal formula for hypertrophy, mainly because hypertrophy is a hand-in-hand process that occurs naturally with resistance training in general. Most coaches who have clients training specifically for aesthetics will often prescribe a rep range of 8 X 10 for three or four sets at 75 to 80 percent 1RM (one rep max), utilizing mostly machine work (i.e., cable flys, leg press, seated dips, etc.). Due to microfilament activities, the proteins and essential amino acids inside the body will be used to increase muscular size.

Building Muscle Strength

Muscular strength is often a desirable goal of training. The best elite athletes will go to great lengths to gain more speed, power, agility, and mobility. With athletes' incredible goals, this is often considered to be the most daunting task of many strength and conditioning coaches. Periodization is broken up into macrocycles of one year, which are broken down to mesocycles of three months, and then carefully examined in separate microcycles of one to three weeks, depending on an athlete's season. Most exercises prescribed are free weighted exercises that open the kinetic chain and force more motor neurons to fire at a higher and faster rate for the athlete to maintain balance while doing the weighted movement. Even still, machines are still commonly used in conjunction with free weight exercises. However, the reason coaches lean towards free weighted exercises is to prepare the athlete for dynamic abilities relative to their respective sport.

The best method of designing a program for strength gains would be to slowly but surely map a periodization plan to the level of 95 to 100 percent 1RM at three to five sets for five to one repetition. This would include power exercises such as bench press, squat, deadlift, hang clean, push jerk, etc. To prevent the athlete from potential injury, it is imperative that the coach em-phasizes form development before loading more and more resistance.

For both hypertrophy and strength, philosophies of increased muscle mass and power stem from a phenomenon called the "overload principle. The overload principle is a training method that requires more and more load for a subsequent set on a particular exercise to the point of exhaustion.

It is important to note that as given by the researcher Fiorilli and team in a 2020 article in *Journal of Sports Sciences and Medicine*: "Training protocols in which the eccentric phase of movement is overloaded, produce greater strength improvements than those in which the load is constant during both the concentric and eccentric phases. Prolonged eccentric exposure can enhance sport performance and prevent injuries." Researcher Cormie and team reported that eccentric training improves concentric force and velocity, enhancing the storage and utilization of elastic energy thus improving muscle performance.

This brings in the next component of overall resistance training called time under tension (TUT), which is defined as the tempo of the repetition itself, quantified in seconds. Coaches will preach slow concentric contractions, and fast eccentric contractions in order to not only elicit speed and power, but to generate heat in the affected area, as well as injury prevention. It is also worth noting that the eccentric contraction will most likely present more of a challenge to complete a one-rep-max (1RM) due to the fact that the athlete will be pushing a load against the combined forces of gravity and the load, making the completion of the 1RM that much more accomplishing.

Weight Loss

As stated earlier, many participants of exercise gravitate towards a fitness center as part of their newfound routine in a desperate attempt at burning fat. Unfortunately, most of these individuals go about their journey the wrong way because they believe that cardio burns fat. This is simply not the case as too much cardio can actually burn away muscle. This happens because it takes away the oxygen that muscles need to generate the necessary heat that burns the adipose tissue (which stores fat). These amounts are quantified in V02 max, which is the maximum amount of oxygen you can utilize during exercise, and they have a maximum input when they are pushed to their absolute limits. The more oxygen your muscles can use, the better your muscles can work, so depleting oxygen through too much cardio often has an opposite effect as desired for someone desiring to burn fat.

Another great determinant to a healthy workout is heart rate. Our heart is responsible for cycling oxygen from the lungs in and out of our bloodstream, and circulating it into all essential systems. The muscles especially need this oxygen to ferment heat production under stress. Therefore, resistance training and weight loss are two sides of one coin when done correctly. As an example, a periodization program for this endeavor would require three sets at 12 to 15 repetitions with weights at 30 to 55 percent of the individual's 1RM. These exercises should be carried out aerobically, emphasizing the importance of reaching the individual's target heart rate range while using resistance training.

Flexibility

Finally, there is also resistance training for flexibility, commonly utilized in rehabilitation settings such as physical therapy and athletic training clinics. This form of resistance training is the most methodical and systematic of all training protocols. More often than not, rehabilitation training is centered around severe injuries that may have required surgery, such as torn ACLs, rotator cuffs, and hip replacements. To prevent muscular degeneration (atrophy), it is the responsibility of the coach to design a program that will aid the rehabilitation of the injured area, without placing too much force on the impingement. Depending on the injury, some exercises that can be used are resistance bands, light calisthenics (body-only exercises), and stretching. For more severe injuries, rehabilitation can be expedited with the use of more advanced technology such as electromagnetic stimulation (EMS), assisted movement braces, cryotherapy, and manual massage therapy. All are designed to be slow in tempo with minimal contraction, and they are used to rebuild neurogenic pathways between the affected limb and the brain as the injured area rebuilds in structure.

Resistance Training for a Successful Body

In the arena of weightlifting, there are still many unanswered questions regarding the kinetics of resistance training and the neurological pathways that elicit such behaviors. Nevertheless, we know an abundant amount of information that gives us the clues for further discovery. So, which form of resistance training is the best? The answer is all of them. One form of exercise for muscles cannot exist over the others, and one cannot dominate over the others. Hormonal regulations serve as "checks and balances" to make sure that each muscle in the human body experiences each and every aspect of the broadened scope of resistance training throughout a person's lifetime. In order to maintain a healthy, functioning body, a successful body, we must consider the balances of all aspects of resistance training to maintain healthy, functional, and efficient muscular tissue that withstands all functional movements on a daily basis, so can experience a long and healthy life.

About the Author

Johnny Spilotro, from Las Vegas, Nevada, has massive ambitions. He earned his Bachelor of Science degree in kinesiology from the University of Nevada Las Vegas while racing competitively in a local NASCAR racing series at the Las Vegas Motor Speedway. With the desire to compete among the best of the best, Johnny's passion for kinesiology stemmed from his own experiences training with elite trainers at several performance clinics throughout Las Vegas Valley. A student of the game, he honed his own knowledge and eventually passed it down to the clients he trains regularly. Johnny's current goals include continuing as a strength and conditioning coach for professional athletes and chasing down his dream of competing in the NASCAR Cup Series.

Email: JohnnySpilotro@Gmail.com
Facebook/Twitter/Instagram:
@JohnnySpilotro
@J_Strength_Conditioning

CHAPTER 28
EAT REAL FOOD

By Denise E. Stegall
CEO & Curator, Living Healthy List
Rochester, Minnesota

Real food doesn't have ingredients, real food is ingredients.
—Jamie Oliver

Deciding what to eat these days can be confusing. Even the word "diet" is confusing—on the one hand, it means starving yourself and eating a very narrow menu; on the other hand (and probably more appealing), a diet is just whatever you eat. By that definition, we all have a diet.

Japanese people traditionally eat fresh fish, vegetables, and rice. If you live around the Mediterranean, traditionally you eat local fish, lots of olive oil, and whatever vegetables and meats are locally grown. In the Nicoya Peninsula of Peru, your traditional diet would consist of locally grown black beans, bananas, plantains, papaya, squash, yams, and homemade corn tortillas. (Is this making you hungry?)

Unfortunately, in the United States, there isn't as much access to locally grown, healthy food. The diet in the US is commonly mass-produced, processed foods, and lots of it. The total caloric intake is often much more than a person needs. We seem to have too many choices in terms of eating and dieting as well—keto, vegetarian, vegan, Paleo. When did healthy eating become so difficult?

Eating Intuitively

The basics of a healthy diet are actually quite simple. Your body needs a mix of proteins, carbohydrates, and fats, plus vitamins and minerals (micronutrients) to sustain a healthy body that feels good, moves well, and functions at its best. Done right, meaning eating more intuitively but not taking in too many calories, your food choices actually protect you against chronic diseases, such as heart disease, diabetes, and cancer. Eating right allows you to do the things you want to do and live a fulfilled life.

Eating a variety of foods, using less salt, sugar, and saturated and trans fats, is essential for a healthy mind, body, and spirit. The foundation of a healthy diet should be simply to eat *real food*, most of the time.

A diet based on **REAL FOOD** may be one of the most important things you can do for your health—body, mind, and spirit. In a nutshell, ***eat real food*** for healthy living and a happy life!

A note here: ***processed foods***, fast food, Twinkies, etc., don't fall into the category of REAL FOOD. The biggest problem with processed foods, in my humble opinion, is that they have way too many calories in them to eat regularly, and they really don't fill you up. Once in a while, maybe, they are okay. If you live on them, they will kill you—literally. By the way, eating at Taco Bell is not eating real food and is not eating intuitively.

What Is Real Food?

Whole foods are as close as possible to the way nature made them. Mostly unprocessed, free of chemical additives, and rich in nutrients. These are the foods people ate prior to the 20th century, when processed, packaged, and ready-to-eat meals became the bulk of the Western diet.

Fruits, vegetables, nuts, seeds, whole grains, legumes, lean meat, poultry, and fish are the staples of a healthy diet of real food. Eating real food is an intuitive lifestyle philosophy, not a diet. "Eat real food" is a very simple concept and not that difficult to adopt.

Eliminating Food Groups? No Way!

When most of us think about eating healthy, what usually comes to mind are all the foods that we have to give up. I'll let you in on a secret: you don't have to completely give up your favorite foods.

While some philosophies suggest otherwise, eating a healthy diet doesn't mean you must eliminate entire categories of food from your plate. That is not intuitive. Each food group provides your body with the nutrition it requires for proper function, and when your body functions well, you feel good.

Improving your health and eating more intuitively could be as easy as swapping unhealthy choices with healthy ones. Over time, you may notice that you have more energy, mental clarity, and possibly a slimmer you. If that's not an incentive to eat real food, I don't know what is.

Rather than eliminating food groups, simply reducing the amount of certain foods may be a better option. Decreasing the amount of meat (all types of meat) you consume improves your health, protects the environment, and reduces the number of animals killed for human consumption. While protein is necessary in your diet, animal protein is high in calories and fat (that's what makes it taste good), which can lead to obesity, cardiovascular disease, and type 2 diabetes.

Do Calories Count?

Again, it is important to choose a healthy diet that will work for you and your family. Instead of eliminating entire food groups, consider selecting the healthiest options from each category. I've included a simple cheat sheet you can find at https://files.constantcontact.com/acb40a7e501/002f2082-3886-4fcc-87a3-852152588dae.pdf to help you get started.

One more thing you need to know—calories do count! There are many thoughts about calorie counting, but at the end of the day, the number of calories you eat versus the calories you burn will have the biggest impact on your health, your weight, and your mindset.

Choose the healthiest foods while staying within your body's unique calorie needs. Too much of a good thing, even fruits and vegetables, can be a bad thing when it comes to your weight. Sounds simple. The right number of calories is different for all of us, so you can use a daily calorie calculator found at https://www.calculator.net/calorie-calculator.html to find out your unique number.

Warning: eating too many calories will cause you to gain weight. Eating too few calories leads to binge eating, feeling tired, weak, and cranky. Fuel your body properly, and it will reward you.

Traffic Light Bites

"Traffic Light Bites" is an easy formula to help you navigate the **Eat Real Food** program. It takes the concept of a traffic light and applies it to what you should and should not eat, and helps you make educated food choices that support your overall health and wellness.

Green Light Foods

Just as a green light at an intersection means it's safe to proceed, green light foods are safe to eat every day. Green light foods are those that are grown and consist of fruits and vegetables, foods you can eat raw, and that are full of the micronutrients your body needs. Additionally, they are low in calories and high in fiber, which fills you up, so you end up eating less.

Green Light Suggestions

- Half of your daily food choices should come from Green Light Foods.
- Aim for a minimum of three servings of vegetables and two servings of fruit every day.
- Eat a rainbow of color. Different colors provide different micronutrients.

Yellow Light Foods

When you're coming up to a light that turns yellow, you need to use caution, and Yellow Light foods warrant you to slow down, too. These foods have more fat, sugar, and calories. They are healthy in that they supply different vitamins, minerals, and nutrients, but extra calories are stored as fat, and we don't want that! Chicken, fish, whole grains, nuts, seeds, whole wheat pasta, sprouted grain breads, low fat dairy, butter, olive oil, and avocados are examples of Yellow Light Foods.

Yellow Light Suggestions

- Eat these foods with some meals, not every meal and not every day.
- These are a necessary part of a healthy diet.
- Avocados are high in calories and fat—even though it is the good fat.

Red Light Foods

You guessed it. Red means STOP! If you want to feel healthy and energetic, you need to stop and reconsider eating these. Red Light Foods include cookies, doughnuts, chips, fried foods, hot dogs, white bread, margarine, soda, deli meats, and pretty much anything in a bag, box, or can. Processed foods like these contain artificial sweeteners, sugar, hydrogenated oils or trans fat, and are loaded with extra fat and calories. I know this sounds daunting. To repeat, pretty much anything in a bag, box, or can is a heavily processed food containing all kinds of extra things that real food does not. It might seem intimidating to try to give up these readily available foods, but with a bit of attention, this lifestyle becomes not only easy, but as you literally feel the difference in your body, the desire to continue eating real foods becomes easy.

Red Light Suggestions

- Consider Red Light Foods a treat to enjoy on occasion.
- Make a different choice or eat a smaller portion. How about a kid's sized burger instead of a double cheeseburger with bacon?
- Avoid margarine made from vegetable oils and trans fats. Not all fats are equal.

The Apple—An Example

To give a visual of Traffic Light Bites, let's look at a simple apple. Conveniently, apples come in green, yellow, and red. An apple in its natural form is a Green Light Food. It provides you with 90 calories, 19 grams of carbohydrates, vitamin C, fiber, and antioxidants, which are really good for you.

Now let's take that apple (plus several more) and make applesauce. First you must remove the skin which eliminates most of the fiber. Then you add sugar to those perfect little apples and cook them, which depletes their nutritious aspects. Now you have a Yellow Light Food. Not bad for you but not as good, either.

Instead of making applesauce, you decide to make an apple pie. Our perfect little apples are now naked without their skin, covered with sugar, butter, flour, and egg, and baked at 350 degrees removing all of the nutritious value and adding about 350 calories per serving. You guessed it—apple pie is a Red

Light food! The good news is that to live a healthy diet you do not need to stop eating apple pie, just lessen the frequency in which you do so.

By now, you understand that eating **Real Food** is the best choice for a healthy, happy lifestyle. The macro- and micronutrients real food provides keep your body working properly, keep your mind clear, and as a bonus, they help you control your weight.

But what happens when we don't make good choices?

Nutrient Deficiency

It's estimated that more than two billion people worldwide are deficient in the vitamins and minerals essential for health, and, yes, most of these people live in underdeveloped countries, but not all. Experts in affluent countries find nutrient deficiencies (malnutrition) in their populations as well. In the United States, there are thousands of people suffering from malnutrition, and most of them don't even know it!

According to one study, just one in ten adults in the United States meets the federal recommendation on fruits and vegetables. Your body doesn't make the micronutrients (vitamins and minerals) that it requires for development, disease prevention, and optimal health, so you must get them from the foods you eat.

When your body doesn't get enough of a micronutrient, you have a deficiency. There are certain medications and certain diseases that can cause malabsorption of nutrients. However, the main culprit in our society is a poor diet full of Red Light Foods. We call this the **S**tandard **A**merican **D**iet or **SAD**.

SAD Story

One summer, a college friend of mine opted to live in Philadelphia rather than head home to his parents' house in the suburbs. Towards the end of the summer, I visited and was aghast at what I saw. His skin looked grey, his eyes sunken, he'd gained a lot of weight, and he was so lethargic he could barely walk three blocks.

When I'd last seen him, three months prior, he was the picture of health. Young, athletic, and energetic, but what I found that day in late August was frightening.

I was studying nutrition in college, so I asked him about his diet.

He handed me the menu of the local restaurant where he ate regularly. Listed were cheesesteaks, burgers, hot dogs, fried egg sandwiches, Cheez Whiz, French fries, and soft drinks. That's it. No vegetables. No fruit. Not one thing that resembled **real food**, and he'd eaten nearly every meal there for three months! I insisted he visit the local clinic where he was diagnosed with malnutrition, even though he had gained a lot of weight.

Why Is This Happening?

We live in a food toxic environment. There's a fast-food restaurant on every corner. Gas stations are filled with snack foods, and supermarkets are overloaded with boxed, bagged, and canned foods that are full of preservatives and fillers. Intended to be a once-in-a-blue-moon, quick, and easy meal for busy families, they have turned into a daily routine for too many people. For many Americans, these highly processed, Red Light Foods have replaced most of the minimally processed, Green Light Foods by about 60 percent.

In fairness, some of these foods are fortified with vitamins and minerals, yet they are still high in calories and low in nutrition. These processed foods represent a health challenge more common in the Western world than we previously thought.

Processed Foods and SAD

What exactly is a processed food and why should you avoid them as much as possible? For starters, processed foods are nutritionally deficient, and they contribute to obesity and the rise of chronic diseases like heart disease, stroke, type 2 diabetes, and certain types of cancer. That should scare you.

But, why are processed foods bad? The answer is that processing compromises the quality of foods and, depending on the degree of processing, removes or completely destroys the nutrition value. No nutrition doesn't mean no calories. It's the exact opposite. Here are a few problems:

- Peeling the outer layer of fruits and vegetables removes nutrients and eliminates fiber.
- Heating or drying foods destroys vitamins and minerals.

The USDA defines a processed food as one that has undergone any changes to its natural state. Any raw agricultural commodity subjected to washing, cleaning, milling, cutting, chopping, heating, pasteurizing, blanching, cooking, canning, freezing, drying, dehydrating, mixing, packaging, or other procedures that alter the food from its natural state is a food that's been processed. This processing may include the adding of artificial colors, flavors, preservatives, nutrients, salt, sugars, and fats. Based on these standards, nearly all foods sold in the supermarket are processed to some degree.

How to Shop to Minimize Processed Foods

When at the supermarket market, select foods from the perimeter of the store. There you'll find the least processed foods, the real foods, like produce, dairy, meat, and fish. If possible, visit your local farmers market or cooperative for locally grown or raised foods. While shopping, also keep in mind the Green Light, Yellow Light, and Red Light Foods to differentiate between the various degrees of food processing.

Green Light Food: Minimally Processed

Green Light foods are minimally processed and are the natural edible parts of plants and animals. They may be slightly altered for preservation but without changing nutrition. Think baby carrots. Pasteurization, refrigeration, pressing, refining, and grinding items like olive oil and whole grain pasta are included in this category.

Yellow Light Food: Processed

Yellow Light foods are processed and have salt, sugar, or fats added to them. Sugar is added to canned fruits, salt to vegetables, and oil to peanut butter to keep it from separating.

Red Light Food: Highly Processed

To live well and feel great, this is the stuff you really need to stay away from *most of the time.* In addition to sugar, salt, and fat, Red Light Foods are highly processed and include artificial colors, flavors, and preservatives that promote shelf stability, preserve texture, and increase palatability. They are also full of calories!

What This Means to You

Are you having trouble getting off the couch or keeping focused at work? The low energy you are experiencing could be the result of the bag of chips you just ate, not lack of ambition.

Do you frequently get sick? A compromised immune system is often a tell-tale sign of a poor diet. If you don't give your body the nutrition it needs, it can't fight off infections.

Do you think as clearly as you used to or struggle to deal with stressful situations? Regularly eating **Real Foods** rich in omega-3 fatty acids, B vitamins, and antioxidants can lead to better mental function and less brain fog. Energy lags, illness, and brain fog all stem from mild nutrient deficiencies. If neglected, this can lead to a list of health conditions and disease.

Make the Change

Are you ready to make the change to a healthier more intuitive way of eating? Apply **Eat Real Food** as your standard and remember **Traffic Light Bites** to help stay on track. I'm a realistic person and understand that even an easy system is hard to stick to 100 percent of the time.

Enter the 80/20 rule. If 80 percent of the time you eat *real food*, then the remaining 20 percent it's okay to enjoy something a little less healthy. What would a birthday be without cake or Thanksgiving without pumpkin pie? Just limit yourself to one slice, okay?

With the 80/20 rule you are following **Eat Real Food** while enjoying your favorite foods and desserts without overindulging. It's a matter of making good choices. One good choice after another leads to a string of choices that gives you everything you need for a healthy, happy, and fulfilling life.

About the Author

As CEO and curator of Living Healthy List, Denise Stegall is a leader who radiates emotional intelligence, positivity, resilience, and a zest for life. Denise has condensed 20 years of experience and study in nutrition, cooking, exercise, and coaching to educate clients on how to live happy, healthy, and productive lives through nutrition and self-empowerment. Her experience in cooking and nutrition delivers a unique perspective on what works (and doesn't work) for most people. Her work revolves around the Living Healthy List Method Pillars of Success: Eat real food, Make good decisions, and be accountable.

As an inspirational thought leader, she is determined to provide Living Healthy List readers with honest, reliable, research-backed content that can be implemented in real life.

Email: Support@livinghealthylist.com
Website: www.livinghealthylist.com
LinkedIn: https://www.linkedin.com/company/living-healthy-list-llc
YouTube: https://www.youtube.com/channel/UCU1u36deqYUYh69OrJjyEXA?
Facebook: https://www.facebook.com/Livinghealthylist/
Instagram: https://www.instagram.com/livinghealthylist/
Twitter: @ListHealthy

CHAPTER 29
PUBLIC SPEAKING, STRESS, AND THE BODY

By Vince Stevenson
Founder, The College of Public Speaking London
London, United Kingdom

It is health that is real wealth—not gold and silver.
—Mahatma Gandhi

When a father's sperm meets a mother's egg, the beauty of human creation begins. Cells divide, and in a short time, you begin to develop what becomes your brain and spinal column. Within there, fibres grow—your nervous system. On the ends of nerve fibres, tiny buds appear—your heart, liver, kidneys, and other essential organs. Your brain connects to every cell in your body via the central nervous system. Your mind and body are connected. What affects one affects the other. An average human being has trillions of cells. Every one of those cells lives an individual life and needs nutrition and care.

How many muscles do you have? Six hundred or 800? My chiropractor tells me that there is just one. As you develop, all the muscle tissue spreads out across your skeleton. Your muscles are all made of the same material. You have shoulder muscles, calf and thigh muscles, and many others. These are just identifiers or categories of muscles. Have you ever had a sports injury, say a dead leg, and had to continue playing with a limp? One muscle becomes incapacitated, so your other muscles try to compensate for it. How do they know? That's easy—they're all connected. Let me reiterate that your mind and body stem from the original single cell. I repeat that every cell connects to the brain via the central nervous system. It means that the status of your body can change in a fraction of a second. Imagine being chased by a sabre-toothed tiger. Your muscles need to react and respond quickly and in an integrated fashion. A signal from the brain triggers a physiological reaction, and those muscle groups must act as one to save your life. It's the same with sexual arousal: a stimulus followed by a physiological reaction. Different organs but the same principle.

Public speaking is both a psychological and physiological discipline. Your mind and body are a phenomenal pairing, indeed the winning combination. Observe Olympic gymnasts, skiers, and Formula 1 drivers. They are exercising microsecond judgements based on visual stimuli. What they're doing is dangerous, and perhaps it's a good thing they don't deliver an accompanying commentary. Yet, the mind and body stretch to the limit. It's not surprising that elite athletes develop into excellent speakers once their sporting careers end. They apply the same meticulous strategies to public speaking that helped them become exceptional athletes.

The human body is engineered for high performance. Although we have yet to master the planet and the universe, humans have mastered their local environment. We have learnt to hunt and survive, to study, to think creatively, to collaborate and to thrive. Humans can travel in outer space and hold our breath for twenty minutes underwater (Stig Severinson—world champion freediver). In terms of difficulty, for most people, public speaking should rank somewhere on the more accessible side of these two extremes, even though many are petrified of it.

Breathing and Oxygen

Humans breathe about 25 thousand to 30 thousand times per day, so this is big business. Our breathing is part of the autonomic nervous system, which means that we breathe even while we are asleep. Because we don't have to think about it, we call it unconscious breathing. When we breathe unconsciously, we utilise up to about 66 percent of our lung capacity. In this section, I want to discuss conscious breathing, where we can access an extra 30 percent of lung capacity/oxygen.

Learning to breathe effectively is your number one tool in managing anxiety. If you don't breathe well, you'll never conquer your speaking demons. The problem is that most people find the breathing solution too simplistic. People are complex and so need complex solutions. Because it's simple, breathing as a founding solution is easily ignored. Let me reiterate this key message—breathing is the key to managing anxiety and public speaking. We need to raise oxygen levels. If there's no fuel in the car, you're not going anywhere. When you breathe consciously, it has a profound impact on your mental acuity and alertness. This improvement is not a surprise. It is inevitable. The more you focus on the task of breathing, the higher the payback.

The most extraordinary change in my speaking performance was when I learned how to breathe consciously. In through the nose, hold it for five seconds, and out slowly through the mouth. This process slows the heart rate down. Lie flat on your bed, arms and legs uncrossed, allow the blood to flow unencumbered. Hold the breath longer and then exhale through tightly pursed lips. I can now hold my breath for up to two minutes, and it slows the heart rate down. It helps me feel calm and in control. But you don't have to lie down to benefit from breathing. The same exercise moments before speaking, while sitting or standing, can have an enormous positive impact.

As we breathe in through the nose, the air, which contains about 20 percent oxygen, gets into our lungs and distributes around the body via our blood vessels. Our brain requires oxygen as do our muscle groups. When oxygen flows freely around the body, all our vital mechanisms are supported.

We know so much more about the human body because health and fitness are prominent modern issues. People have created remarkable tools, like FMRI scanners, so we can observe the distribution of oxygen in the brain in real-time. We know that when we breathe in deeply, our blood vessels dilate. This improves blood flow and creates a greater throughput of oxygen around the brain and body. We can see which parts of the brain get stimulated through oxygen flow.

As a young footballer, they told me to breathe in through the nose and exhale through the mouth. When I asked why, the best answer I received was that "it seems to work." These days, the scientific proof is compelling.

The Vagus Nerve

The vagus nerve is about one metre long, and it's the longest nerve in the body. It gets its name from the word vagabond, meaning a wanderer. It wanders through the neck, the heart and lungs, the diaphragm, and down through our intestines and into our reproductive organs. There is a right and left vagus nerve, though it's often discussed in the singular. The vagus nerve is important because it is one of the most prominent ways we feel stress in our body.

The nervous system divides into two halves. First is the "fight or flight", the stress system, known as the sympathetic nervous system. The second is known as "rest and digest", and it is the parasympathetic nervous system.

Stress causes a presence of adrenaline in the blood, which kickstarts the sympathetic nervous system. Your muscles contract, the heart beats faster, and your blood pressure can remain high over long periods. Chronic stress created by a build-up of cortisol can cause a lack of productivity, followed by absentee-ism, and a general sense of burn out. At this point, you are more susceptible to strokes and heart attacks. Though mild stress is normal, if you think stress is bad for your health, it can be a killer. Listen to your body and slow down if needed.

Cortisol is a survival hormone. You have to fight the sabre-toothed tiger or run. (Best run actually). Yet, thought-induced anxiety has the same physi-ological impact and symptoms. Social anxiety, the pressure at work, anything that creates stress continues and accumulates, resulting in digestive problems. It also damages the immune system because while your brain is fighting on one front, nothing is happening on the other side to restore the balance of your cells and muscles. Food digestion and nutrient levels diminish. Over an extended period, you can become unhealthy.

The opposite of fight-or-flight is the rest-and-digest phenomenon, which is linked to the parasympathetic nervous system. There are specific chemicals within our body that are linked to the parasympathetic nervous system. They are serotonin, which is a neurotransmitter associated with happiness and well-being, and dopamine, a neurotransmitter associated with reward-motivated behaviour.

In life, we need a balance. You shouldn't be too stressed or too relaxed either. But it's important to be challenged in our studies, careers, and sporting activities. Without challenge, you'll never know the full extent of the pleasures of achievement, and you'll never become resilient.

Modern humans tend to operate more on the stressed "fight-or-flight" side because of the mental stimuli we receive—too many tasks and not enough time. We seem to always be chasing our tail. When you take a pause and sense that you're too busy, there is something very easy you can do. Simply breathe slowly, hold your breath, and exhale slowly, and you tap directly into the para-sympathetic nervous system. It helps to lower the heart rate and helps you stay focused. Almost immediately, you can feel the shift of your mind arriving in that more relaxed place.

And for a great tip, just remember what world champion freediver Stig Severinson says that the nose is for breathing and the mouth is for eating.

Don't be fooled by the simplicity of breathing. It's highly efficient. How could anything so simple be so beneficial?

As an exercise in breathing, try 1:2 breathing: inhale through the nose for five seconds and then exhale for ten seconds. The double exhale sends the signal to slow down the heart. Try and make the sound of a sigh as you exhale. Controlled respiration is essential for this process. Also, try to relax the jaw as we tend to hold a lot of emotional tension there. Breathing is a neurophysiological technique, and it's the cornerstone of public speaking and reducing general stress. If you're not breathing effectively, you'll never have the fuel, or the poise, required to hit the speaking heights.

Nitric Oxide (Not Nitrous Oxide)

Nitric oxide is a naturally occurring molecule of gas in your body. Its significance in restoring a healthy balance in the cells is well documented. In 1992, nitric oxide was awarded the "Molecule of the Year" award, and in 1998, Furchgott, Ignarro, and Murad won the Nobel Prize in Medicine and Physiology for discovering nitric oxide as a signalling molecule in the cardiovascular system.

How does nitric oxide work?

The endothelium is the lining of the blood cells and is a massive spatially distributed organ in the body (on average 60 thousand to 100 thousand miles long) and one cell thick. It's vital for distributing blood and oxygen around your brain, tissues, and organs. The primary cause of cardiovascular disease is a build-up of plaques within the artery walls. In a healthy artery, the blood flow is smooth and free, and that's how you want to keep it. If the artery hardens by plaque, it's less flexible and less effective. Relaxation is essential for life generally as well as public speaking. It's so much easier to relax when your body is working for you rather than against you. Nitric oxide is liberated from the amino acid l-arginine, which is encouraged by selective foods (see below) and stimulated by moderate exercise and breathing relaxation techniques. There's every reason to take advantage of its curative attributes. Over 100 thousand studies into nitric oxide tell us of its importance in cellular activities where it:

- Improves communication between brain cells
- Assists in gastric efficacy

- Regulates blood pressure by dilating arteries (allows greater relaxation)
- Assists the immune system to kill bacteria
- Reverses erectile dysfunction
- Reduces inflammation
- Improves sleep quality
- Increases your recognition of sense (i.e., smell)
- Increases endurance and strength (bodybuilders/athletes love it)

Nitric oxide naturally accumulates in your nasal cavity as well as through-out the endothelium. When we breathe in and hold the breath, this incredible gas redistributes around your body through the cardiovascular system. It penetrates the central nervous system and delivers its healing powers to your body's 30 to 50 trillion cells. To access this incredible molecule, all you need to do is breathe in through the nose and hold it and let it do its work. Once you reach the age of 40, your body begins to produce less nitric oxide, which is in line with the ageing process. So, we need to access and make the most of it via deep breathing and yoga, Pilates, or other similar exercises.

Green-leafed vegetables like spinach and kale also help generate a healthy supply of nitric oxide as do meat (particularly animal organs), walnuts, beets, garlic, onions, cayenne pepper, dark chocolate, shrimp, oranges, pomegranates, and cranberries (all in moderation).

For many years, yoga, meditation, and the Eastern traditions were frowned upon in Western scientific communities as they lacked scientific verification. Since 1998, however, there is a massive volume of research into the benefits of nitric oxide and meditative practices that help generate it. Nitric oxide is free to use. All you need is to make a choice and start to access the benefits. Everything about nitric oxide is a winner.

Sleep: Another Natural Healer

If you work in a high-pressure job and you find public speaking an awkward bolt-on to your daily duties, a lack of sleep is the last thing you need. Sleep has a direct impact on your mood, motivation, and general performance. It's good for the brain, memory, and cognition, and it's good for your personal and working relationships. Giving a presentation while exhausted is unhealthy for you and your reputation, and it's a low-quality experience for the audience. Those who are tired, look and sound tired. If you're tired and grumpy, you don't want to be in front of a class or the board of directors answering questions. When you're in the wrong frame of mind, your presentation will NOT be as good as it could be. A good night's sleep and a planned regime is a significant booster of performance in speaking and many other areas that require you to be at your best.

When I am working in London, I have a strict routine. I am in bed before 10:30 pm, and my alarm rings at 6:50 am. I do 10 minutes of conscious breathing to start the day. I leave home at 7:50 and take the 8:00 am train, which, allowing for delays and cancellations, should see me in class for 9:30 am. Having that sacred ritual gives me a focus and a sense of certainty, which is good for confidence. As a trainer, the worst thing is to arrive late for class, leaving a large group of students waiting. Life can be stressful enough without succumbing to bad planning. Having a coherent regime means I get a good night's sleep knowing that I am aware of the constants and managing the variables the best I can (an old programmer's joke).

Exercise and Relaxation

Going to the gym is not everybody's idea of fun. Neither is it everybody's idea of exercise. I am not keen on the gym myself although, in the autumn and winter, that's where you will find me six to seven hours per week. I have a set regime, a flexible contract with myself and my family that I attend the gym for an hour on days when I do not have clients or classes.

For me, a great exercise is a walk in the park, taking in the fresh air and the greenery. In the spring and summer, my family will go for a country walk for a few hours, and then the reward is a pub lunch. Fresh air, pretty landscapes, and a reasonable walking pace are all that your body needs to feel refreshed and invigorated. Contact with nature is a great motivator. Exercise releases endorphins and inhibits pain. Runners/athletes/gym-goers feel euphoric highs like other naturally occurring opioids, and dopamine, the reward hormone, also provides a temporary lift. Cortisol, the stress hormone, is washed from your system. Exercise is one of the best things for you.

If, like me, you spend most of your life in an air-conditioned office or a centrally heated flat, the wide-open spaces are calling you for a good reason. Before marriage, most summers I would go on a walking tour to the Lake District. In 1995, I spent five months hiking in South and Central America. I have never been happier than walking in beautiful landscapes, not knowing what I'd find over the next hill.

Why is this important for speakers? I find walking inspiring. It invokes ideas and takes you out of home and office. Everything looks possible when you're in the middle of nowhere on a sunny day, and all you can hear is a faint breeze or the gurgling of a stream. We experience clarity of thought and connection with the landscape. We recognise that it's the simplest pleasures in life that offer the most significant rewards.

For those who prefer the gym, why not try an extended session? Do your usual routine and then add a mix of stretching and breathing exercises. Don't forget to remain hydrated in the gym. Drink water between exercises and warm-up for each activity. If you haven't exercised for some years, have a consultation with your doctor. For those individuals who find sleeping hard, this one activity—conscious breathing—will have a significant impact on all aspects of your life.

We take weekend walks in the countryside. So, how about a walk to the park at lunchtime? Even in big city centres, you'll find parks with lawns and benches. Take some time out of the office and breathe. Slow your heart rate down and relax. Looking after your health is the best investment in your future. Operating with a clear mind is invaluable. Speaking with clarity is precious. And all of these things are within your grasp.

About the Author

Vince Stevenson is a speaker, trainer, author, and CEO of the College of Public Speaking London, one of the UK's leading public speaking, management, and leadership development organisations. As an athletic young man, Vince had a huge interest in physiology, psychology, nutrition, health, and well-being. Vince is the author of *The Fear Doctor* and *Anxiety Quick Wins*, and a co-author of *The Successful Mind*, all available on Amazon. Vince is also the author of his South America historical memoir entitled, *The Truck 1995*. Five months on the road from Ushuaia, Argentina to Mexico City.

Email: vince@collegeofpublicspeaking.co.uk
Website: https://www.collegeofpublicspeaking.co.uk/about-us/vince-stevenson

CHAPTER 30

KEEPING IT SIMPLE: PRACTICAL ADVICE FOR A HEALTHIER LIFE

By Fozi Stinson
Holistic Pain Management Coach, Nutritionist
Mississauga, Ontario, Canada

We carry inside us the wonders we seek outside us.
—Rumi

We all have that voice in our head that parrots all the health advice we've heard our entire life. The one we likely don't listen to because we already know what it's saying: drink more water, eat the rainbow, and for the love of all that's good in the world, hop on the treadmill before the week is over. That voice may be nagging and lack sympathy for the struggles of day-to-day existence, but its heart is in the right place. Much like our conscience, it's trying to tell us something we need to hear. Sometimes, rather than fighting or suppressing it, we need to look at how we can realistically integrate its advice into our routines.

Modern life makes it hard to achieve every aspect of health to perfection; simply adjusting our standards from 100 percent to 90 percent can take the pressure off while still ensuring we are living a life that fulfills our mental and physical needs. Most people have a vague idea of how a healthy lifestyle should look, but they are still a little fuzzy on why, what, and how.

There is one thing we can all agree on though: health and wellness are crucial elements of life. Without a sense of physical and spiritual well-being, the experience of life is less enjoyable, and the activities of day-to-day life that we could all enjoy are sapped of their value. Even though we often disregard the importance of nourishing our bodies and spirit, a healthy body that you feel good in contributes to a healthy mindset, and vice versa.

When it comes to choosing habits to incorporate into your lifestyle, there are certainly some to avoid, which we have all been warned of at length throughout our lives. On the other hand, we are not as often advised on what to seek out, and when we are, it is usually with the mindset of avoiding a health risk, rather than encouraging an actively positive bodily state. Below you will find both types of advice: habits to avoid and routines to actively cultivate your physical and mental well-being.

Food and Nutrition

Below are two broader principles of nutrition that you can fall back on. A healthy diet should include:

- Higher intakes of vegetables and fruits, whole grains, fat-free or low-fat dairy, seafood, legumes, and nuts
- Lower intakes of meats (especially processed meats and processed poultry), sugar-sweetened foods (particularly beverages), and refined grains

Eating fruit and vegetables can also increase your life expectancy. A 2017 review of studies published by BMJ company found an average five percent reduction in risk of mortality from all causes with each serving of fruit or vegetables eaten, up to five servings per day. Never underestimate the importance of eating the full rainbow. If you cook, you will have to buy groceries anyway, so sneak in as many colors of fruits and veggies as you can.

If you are overweight or obese, shedding excess pounds is another way to prevent disease or manage conditions you already have, such as diabetes, arthritis, or high blood pressure. According to the National Institutes Health (NIH), in America, two out of three adults and one in six children are at least overweight. If you are experiencing this issue, rest assured that you are not the only one to blame. We are marketed massive portions of greasy and fatty food daily. Millions of people are now victims of consumer culture, and you are *not* alone. That said, you are also not alone in recognizing the genuine health risks and wanting to take action.

Luckily, there is no shortage of ways you can do precisely that. While depriving yourself of food for long periods is never a good idea, intermittently fasting is an excellent way to reduce your overall food intake. You can do this by either fasting all day on selected days (a typical ratio is fasting two out of every seven days) or by fasting for a certain number of hours per day (a popular strategy is to consume food only between 12 noon and 8 pm). While you should always be wary of overeating on non-fasting days, generally, these regimens are more likely to help than hinder you on your optimal health and weight-loss journey.

If the micro-fasting from 8 pm through the next day's lunch isn't your cup of tea, eating a high-protein breakfast is another tried-and-true method of losing weight, and it is usually quite easy to implement. Protein can help decrease the hunger hormone known as ghrelin and contribute to a rise in chemicals within the body that promote feelings of fullness, such as cholecystokinin. The hormonal effects of a high-protein breakfast can last for several hours, so this idea has a tremendous effort-to-reward ratio. If you are at a loss for what to eat other than bread and butter, great breakfast choices include oats, eggs, nuts, seed butter, chia seeds, and sardines.

As with most aspects of health, adopting a meditative outlook can inspire huge benefits. If you commit to eating and chewing slowly, you will find that it is easier to recognize when you are starting to get full. In a similar vein, try to avoid the distraction of your phone or the television while you eat. These practices will help you to focus on the nourishment in front of you, helping you cultivate a deep appreciation for food, rather than the entitled attitude to which many of us have grown accustomed. Appreciating your food has the natural consequence of helping you understand your body; after all, we are what we eat.

Remember: you can make any improvements or changes you need to in stages. There's no need to try to tackle every aspect of your health all at once. Pick one part of your health you want to focus on and devote a week to it. You might start an exercise program, find out which screening tests you're due for and make appointments for them, making a small change or two to your diet, or take steps to kick the habit if you're a smoker.

Substances: Dos and Don'ts

We all know that smoking has detrimental health effects. The list of diseases and cancers attributed to smoking is long, but sometimes long-range concerns prompt less change than immediate concerns. Immediate problems can include shortness of breath, discolored teeth, and irritability.

Alcohol should be consumed only in moderation, and for many people, not at all. Some harmful health effects of alcohol include higher risks of disease and alcohol poisoning. Alcohol is known to promote violence, both against the self and against others. It can cause depression and anxiety, which is also toxic to relationships. Long-term alcohol use can pose a severe threat to the health of your liver, whether in the form of cirrhosis or liver failure.

At the same time, moderate quantities of alcohol can have their benefits. Alcohol has a bad reputation due to how harmful it can be in excess, but if you value the experience of controlled alcohol use, being realistic about its benefits is the first step to integrating it into your lifestyle. For women, the recommendation is one drink a day or less; for men, two. This is on account of not only differences in body size, but also differences in body fat content and the fact that women have less ADH, the enzyme that breaks down alcohol.

And yet, the question remains: if not alcohol, what fluids should you be consuming? As you may already know, you can't go wrong with water. However, you may not be aware of the many benefits to be reaped from drinking water consistently throughout the day. Because it seems like such an obvious and readily available beverage, many of us neglect to prioritize water consumption. Though there is no universally accepted daily quantity of water that we should drink, we know that water makes up 60 percent of our bodies, and so it's arguably an essential part of our diets. It has its uses as a beauty product as well: without proper hydration, our skin is more likely to wrinkle and develop disorders.

If you need some visuals to help you appreciate the full range of benefits water has to offer, here are a few descriptions of its functions within the body. Our joints need lubrication, and the cartilage found in our joints contains about 80 percent water. Without water, our joints can become less shock-resistant and cause us pain. Blood, for another example, is over 90 percent water, and it's necessary to transport oxygen all around our bodies. We need pressure in our veins to keep blood cycling through our bodies at a healthy rate.

These lifestyle behaviors can go a long way in helping you live a long, healthy life. But we know that living goes beyond good physical health; mental, social, and spiritual health are equally important. Practicing stress management, developing a passion or hobby, and pampering yourself at times should be high on your to-do list. Self-care is an ever-growing pop culture phenomenon, but it can go much deeper than bubble baths and candles. Self-care is listening to your body and its needs; it also means knowing when to tell yourself no. It's listening to your muscles when they need a stretch, and even when they need a rest. It's listening to your sugar cravings but opting to consume nuts or grains instead for the time being.

Building healthy eating habits can protect your health, prevent disease, and minimize the severity of conditions you already have. It is one of the fundamental building blocks of health; before you consider what activities to partake in or committing to a work schedule, you would be wise to take inventory of your diet and eliminate consumption of any foods that don't make you feel your best.

Resting the Body and Mind

Physical health is the first key to living a life of balance. You can help your physical body thrive in several ways. It is one of the greatest ironies of life that we often sacrifice sleep, which is essential to our functioning in the world, to achieve more. While there exist effective remedies for sleepless nights (coffee, anyone?), there truly is no replacement for a good night's sleep. That's because our body is hard at work repairing and adjusting as we slumber. A lack of sleep can produce a diabetic-like state in the body, even if we are otherwise healthy. Sleep occurs in cycles that include both deep sleep and rapid eye movement (REM), ideally four to five times over before we wake up. It is a great habit to get into bed early, so our body can take all the time it needs to perform these cycles. Besides, if we wake up in the quieter hours of the morning, we will feel remarkably refreshed and ready to start the day.

When you are well-rested, you will feel it in every part of your body and feel empowered to make decisions from a feeling of abundance, rather than scarcity. Meditation, something of a panacea for stress-induced conditions, is beneficial as an antidote to insomnia. Meditation has been proven to improve mental state as well as ease physical pain. There is a wide selection of meditation apps to ease you into the process if you are unsure where to start.

As a rule, implementing any lifestyle change is far from easy. If you are finding the idea of altering your normal behaviors overwhelming, try devoting a few days out of the week to cultivating awareness of one issue and how it has been affecting your life. Allow yourself to engage in activities that clear your mind. This might look like walking in the park, putting on calm music and assuming a restful position, or attending a mindfulness-based yoga class. Try to become aware of the deeper desires that are motivating you to seek better health, such as being able to show up for your family or engage in physical activities you've been missing. While the thought of implementing a healthier lifestyle may be intimidating, once you start, you just might find that it is not only easier than you think, but that you begin to love the positive changes not only in your physical body, but in your whole life.

About the Author

Fozi Stinson is passionate about your health and wellness. As a pain management coach, nutritionist, yoga instructor, Reiki master, and CBT counselor, she is confident she can help you along your healing journey, not just because she strongly believes in the natural health products and methods she offers, but because she has been where you are.

Before starting on the path of natural health and wellness, Fozi suffered from fibromyalgia, severe osteoarthritis, and neuropathic pain. For years she struggled to overcome physical and emotional suffering using traditional methods. However, a combination of nutrition, whole food supplements, yoga, meditation, and Reiki allowed her to better be able to understand her own body and mind, and ultimately harness the healing powers within and around her. Since discovering and mastering these methods, Fozi has enjoyed improved physical and mental health allowing her to live life better, and her occupation is now passing this information on to help others and improve their lives.

Email: fozistinson@gmail.com
Website: https://painreliefone.com/

CHAPTER 31

HYPNOSIS FOR PERMANENT WEIGHT LOSS

By Leslie M. Thornton
Podcast Host, Hypnosis for Permanent Weight Loss
Albany, New York

In silence there is beauty, wisdom, and the answer.
—Unknown

My whole life I thought I had to be strong. I thought it wasn't okay to cry, or feel angry, or be afraid. I'm still not okay showing I'm afraid, and I'm still not totally comfortable letting anyone know I'm not fine. But what is fine, really? How come sometimes I feel okay and sometimes I feel angry? And why does it cause me to eat?

For over three decades that I've lived thus far, I have been on a never-ending journey of feeling pain and fixing the bad feelings. Growing up, I was the middle child of four girls. I remember my dad saying one night at dinner, when the whole house was emotionally falling apart, "I just look at Leslie and if she's okay, I know that I can remain calm." I took on being the emotional rock in my family, which was really hard. By the time I was 8 years old, extra weight started to accumulate on my body. And rather than being supported to express my feelings and emotions, I was instructed on how to control my weight with socially available rules about calories in and calories out, Weight Watchers, etc. How 21st century, right? And this began the very real process of my learning to numb myself through eating (which felt like control but was fake), and it was the start of my internal disaster.

On the flip side, being brought up that way had a lot of perks. Currently, as a leader and as a professional, I am a force to be reckoned with. You'd never know I was scared or nervous. I can always make anyone, and everyone, feel safe and at home and taken care of. I spent four years as a registered nurse in the neuro and surgical ICU and kidney transplant unit taking care of patients day after day.

In my early 20s, I traveled around the world, living in Bali, Thailand, Australia, and New Zealand. I meditated twice a day after being exceptionally and intimately trained in Tantric meditation by a 70-year-old, former hippy, and science college professor. During my travels, I eliminated all "feeling substances" like alcohol, sugar, flour, caffeine, marijuana, and even unnecessary snacking. For three straight years, I did this almost perfectly. I proved to myself, and to others, that I could still be happy and fulfilled without the added numbing effects of these substances. I have proven that I can lose and maintain a whole bunch of weight in an extremely controlled manner by taking out certain food groups, like dairy and gluten. I have proven that I can say no when repeatedly offered food or drinks. I could go out and party with the digital nomad community I was a part of every other night, dancing the night away, without drinking. My peers would approach me and ask me, "How do you do it? You're still having just as much fun, maybe even more fun than anyone else."

But when it comes to my personal life, my relationship with my family, my friends, and my health? Well, I have had to work much, much harder. In fact, all my clients are super successful in their careers, but they can't figure out why they have so much trouble with food and relationships, despite their professional success. "What's wrong with me?" they ask. There IS a direct correlation between depression and not feeling able to ask for help. Basically, when you're programmed not to be weak, and to internalize all your emotions, you feel you don't have permission to ask for help. I remember being afraid that if I did, nobody would be able to trust me with their feelings again or be able to ask me for help. Maybe they'd even abandon me or think I was a failure. Scary! So, I had to find a different way to cope with stress and anxiety, and I pretty quickly returned to food and alcohol.

So, what happens when you stop numbing? What happens when you take away the diet plan, the food rules, the calories in and calories out? What happens when you allow yourself to feel vulnerable and scared? What happens when you start eating and can't stop? What happens when there are no crutches for emotional support anymore? It is absolutely terrifying, actually. But when you have a guide to help you feel and know that it is safe to feel, it's a game-changer.

You Must Feel Your Pain

Probably one of the scariest things my weight-loss clients have to do is share their shame and experience their feelings in a vulnerable way. There's so much shame about being so obsessed with body image and weight and food because "no one understands" that madness. But pretending like it's not there only makes it worse. We must share the shame, ask for help, and make a change, a radical change.

Let's be real. No one wants to sit in a negative feeling at all. It feels awful. And, the only way to get to the other side is through. The only way change can happen is if you understand the source of the pain and feel that and move through that. But you definitely need a guide. I know I did. I was super scared to feel my pain and emotions. It was foreign territory for me, and I have seen it is the same for all my clients. You quite literally feel like you're going to die having to sit and not numb in some way, shape, or form. Having a guide or a coach helps. Understanding that feelings are just temporary and that they pass after just 30 seconds of attention, 30 seconds of breathing and noticing, and sometimes adding some mindful technique, is a game-changer.

Even right now, I invite you to close your eyes, take a breath, and mentally scan your body. Right now, you have some source of stress or anxiety that you can feel as a difference of energy and temperature in your body. Take a deep breath right now. Breathe into that sensation of stress or anxiety in your body. Ask: *what would this sensation say if it had a voice? If this sensation had something it was scared of or something it did not want to happen, what would that be?* Its response is usually in a third grader's mentality, as this is when the subconscious mind's blueprint is laid out. So the response may be something like, *I'm scared. I hate this. It's not fair. Nobody likes me. Everybody hates me. Guess I'll go eat worms!* Something exactly like that. It can sound silly but trust it. Whatever phrase comes up will have the same sound as the vibration in your body, and it is exactly what you want to have happen no matter what that is. It takes a little practice, but it's very effective.

I remember when I found hypnosis for permanent weight loss in 2011. It was revolutionary for me. I was super anxious at parties or buffets and was scared to leave the house without a backpack full of food. Most of all, I was super afraid of gaining weight. And then I listened to a recording of a hypnosis session I had previously done, and I became totally at peace in all those situations. Seriously, just like that. I had to do a lot of pre-work and maintenance work thereafter, but it started me on my journey of being able to control my mind and change the way I was feeling that gave me completely different results. I was no longer feeling panicked about gaining weight because inner peace is all I ever really wanted, and I found it.

I remember, not too long ago, hearing about the concept of unconditional love. "I am worthy and deserving of experiencing unconditional love" was a mantra I often heard. But what does unconditional love actually mean? What is it like to feel unconditional love? At the root, I think it is what we're all craving. Freedom to be loved and accepted just as we are, imperfections and all. All parts of ourselves: happy, sad, anxious, depressed, miserable, all want to be loved unconditionally. Only love comes back. What would that be like? All over and everywhere? No negative reactions, no people getting mad. What would it be like to be all the good and bad parts of yourself with only getting love back? To some, that may seem easy, but if you're stuck in food prison, you don't have that because you're not at peace with this part of yourself yet. I get that, and it doesn't have to be that way ... at all. But you have to ask for help and make a change. You'll hear me say that a hundred times on my podcast because it's absolutely true. The truth will set you free.

In my story, I traveled away from my family for two years, as far away around the world as I could go, just to try to get my family to love and accept me. I also went there to try to find a man brave enough for me. I traveled to develop a business plan that would grow because people would pay attention to me and how far away I had traveled. The point is that I went to extreme measures to get exactly what I wanted, which included world travel.

I didn't know that was happening at the time, but that became apparent when I still wasn't finding the kind of man I wanted to marry, or the kind of business success I wanted to have, or the family relationships and body acceptance that I desired. And I got to the end of my rope, feeling helpless about all of the things I was searching for and not getting.

Do you want to know the only thing that made a difference for me? Coaching.

Investing in myself was the best thing I did for myself. Getting coached by relationship experts, spiritual advisors, business coaches, and health coaches was what made the real difference for me. There was no better way for me to rewire my subconscious mind than to go within, feel my emotions, get clarity on exactly what I wanted, and then get strategic coaching from others who had already done the same as I wanted to do. I was able to take from their experiences and apply what I learned in a way that worked for me in my own life.

Another thing that made a difference for me was in learning how to truly embrace myself in my authentic truth, happiness, and well-being. I focused on how relationships, body, health, happiness, and lifestyle resonated with ME. Who am I beyond my parents, beyond what I had always known or had been exposed to? Who am I beyond all of what I thought could have been possible? And you know what? My parents are finally starting to see and believe what I am capable of, and I have 100 percent stopped trying to explain or prove or justify myself to anyone. Some people never master that. These people are innocent yet hold caustic childhood wounds.

I have recently started to take 100 percent responsibility for who I am, what I want, and I am never willing to take no for an answer. I know how to set boundaries without making others feel bad. I know how to take care of my energy and my sacred space. I know where to go and what I need in any given feeling that I have in my body to make me truly feel nourished and feel better, so I can keep taking action faster, and so I can make a bigger difference for people wherever I go. It is absolutely insane and wonderful.

Currently I am 5 feet, 2 inches tall, and I weigh 160 pounds. I have been this weight for one year consistently. I have maintained this weight with absolutely no food rules or diets or programs. Simply by saying yes to my desires and doing what I feel will make me feel great next (even if that sometimes includes alcohol or sweets). The freedom within is absolutely priceless, and the anxiety over my weight has disappeared.

Although I am not the model of thinness, I am comfortable with my weight. The transition into my current size-ten body was one of the most painful experiences I have ever gone through. It forced me to face ultimate fears of rejection and abandonment from my very weight-conscious family and from friends. I had to face the fear of gaining weight itself, the fear that I would never attract a mate. Basically, all fears of being able to survive as a potentially fat and ugly woman banned from society for her failures and apparent shortcomings.

But guess what? None of those fears came true. What happened instead was the exact opposite. I have a thriving, six-figure coaching business, I have attracted a relationship with a beautiful man who models unconditional love.

My relationships with my friends and family are better than ever, and my health is top-notch without any obsession. The results of learning how to be at peace and at home in my body and for myself completely changed my life and gave me all I ever wanted without ever having to leave home. In fact, I am still home now, happy as a clam, doing what I love … helping YOU believe in your successful body as well.

If I were still anxious and preoccupied with my weight, I wouldn't be able to have the presence and peace of mind to take care of others and myself at the capacity I have today. I have an extremely successful podcast, and each and every day, people are once and for all getting free from the food and weight obsession, permanently, for good. And it can be you IF you start by taking action right now.

About the Author

Leslie M. Thornton is a female entrepreneur and transformational leader in the coaching and consciousness industry. She is an NLP practitioner and founder of Hypnosis for Permanent Weight Loss and host of the *Hypnosis for Permanent Weight Loss* podcast. Leslie is a registered nurse with professional certifications and training in coaching and cutting-edge subconscious mind modalities, tools that allow for the permanent weight-loss experience and overall life satisfaction of the individuals and groups she professionally coaches. If you want to become permanently free from anxiety over your weight, contact Leslie today, right now. Do not wait. You've been waiting long enough.

Email: leslie@lesliemthornton.com
Website: www.weightlossalbany.com

CHAPTER 32

YOUR BODY: THE MOST VALUABLE MACHINE

By David H. Wallis, M.D.
Family & Sports Medicine, Team Physician, Ironman Competitor
Hermosa Beach, California

Thirst was made for water; inquiry for truth.
—C.S. Lewis

Confession: I am the guy who throws away the instructions without reading them. That is my step one for all projects. Building furniture, setting up a computer, any power tool in the garage—I like to "just figure it out." Confession #2: I have had to dejectedly retrieve said discarded instructions from the trash on more than one occasion.

But I am also the guy who knows that the more complex, the longer-lasting, and the more dire the consequences of screwing it up, the more important we get it right in the first place. When it comes to our body, we need to read the manual—our manual. And while the context in which you live today probably bears little resemblance to the one our species was designed to survive many thousand years ago, we need to remember that our genetics and biology have changed very little since then.

Intelligent people will debate whether the very survival of our species hinged upon successfully implementing the hunter/gatherer lifestyle by which we evolved, or whether we were designed exactly with that means of survival in mind. Regardless, the fact is that the hunter/gatherer lifestyle is completely foreign to our current lives—and our bodies show and feel it. Likewise, there are many more functions, both simple and complex, that we were designed for, but which we have largely discarded, lost sight of, or never developed to their potential. We must do better. We need to start paying attention to, and analyzing, what we know about the human condition, so we can learn from this brilliant design and adapt these lessons to modern-day society.

Our body is a magnificent machine, but we often harm and/or demean it by treating it as a plaything. Though it works amazingly well despite our neglect, in order to optimize this amazing instrument, we need to study the owner's manual. Using a tool in ways other than intended—for example, using a kitchen knife as a screwdriver or using a chisel to open a paint can—may get the job done, but certainly compromises both the efficiency of the task and lifespan of the tool. Properly using and caring for something as complex as our body is easier said than done, but so much more important.

The relative simplicity of a child's toy enables the Christmas Eve assembly of the toy, with or without the instructions. If the toy doesn't work, the only thing that usually gets hurt is the parent's pride. But up the ante to a Ferrari, and people suddenly decide they should at least save the owner's manual in the glove box. They may not read it cover to cover, but the stakes are higher. And if you are talking about a Formula 1 race car, you add in a whole team of professionals whose very careers have been spent studying optimal design and engineering—for the engine, the suspension, the computer system, and their integration with each other—which are all critical to keep the car performing optimally. Step up the technology even more and look at a fighter jet or space-craft, and the "owner's manual" involves thousands of brilliant minds, millions of pages of documents, billions of lines of code, etc.

So then why do we, equipped with the human body as our ultimate ma-chine—a machine that makes the most complex spacecraft or supercomputer look like a simple toy under the proverbial Christmas tree—fail to pay atten-tion to the manual? I dispute any claim that there is no manual. We have the wisdom of millennia and billions of others to learn from, but we choose not to. We fail to consider how our body was designed; we fail to study best practices for our species or ourselves; we fail to implement lessons already learned and are doomed to make the same mistakes again and compound our consequences. We fail to pursue our own optimization, even when both the quantity and quality of our very life depend on it.

To say we fail at all these things may not be completely fair. To be fair, not everyone is interested in figuring it out. Some don't believe that they can. Some realize how important it is. Some are so distracted with things of the world that they never allocate the bandwidth to develop themselves. All of us at times succumb to the path of least resistance, not choosing to swim upstream for the moment and letting entropy set in. In the long run, however, this is not without consequence.

The intricacies of the machine that we inhabit—body, mind, and spirit—may be beyond our ability to fully comprehend, but much can be learned and adopted to optimize them. While it is absurd to ignore the instructions for a fighter jet and just try to "figure it out," with something even more complex and important, we ignore the instructions and think we can just figure it out like an Ikea towel rack. In doing so, we demean our true potential and the gift of this marvelous machine.

It's understandable why we do this. After all, we were simply born inhabiting these bodies and have tried to "figure it out" from day one with, or in spite of, the teachings of parents, siblings, teachers, peers, religious guides, physicians, and the media. We all lifehack our way through, and depending on your upbringing and your situation, you could justifiably come to some pretty wild conclusions about how you are "supposed" to work. In today's age of information overload, you can feed your confirmation bias by finding anything you want online, so what you read often bolsters whatever potentially misguided beliefs you already have. Combined with our unfounded and entitled assumption that everything "should" work just right, we tend to focus on the 0.0001 percent of things that go wrong instead of the 99.9999 percent that go right with our bodies every day.

I am going to give you a glimpse of several different angles to evaluate your own body, the "machine" you inhabit. Think of these angles as sections in your "owner's manual." While there are dozens of components that would qualify as major section headings in an owner's manual for the human body, in this chapter, I'm only going to highlight just a few. While we all share many parts of this owner's manual due to shared biological origins, we are also custom models with unique combinations of millions of individual options, thanks to our DNA, our upbringing, other environmental factors, etc. As such, I encourage you to continue developing your own manual further by being curious, asking questions, and compiling notes on how you optimally operate.

I am a physician. As such, I would not fault you for expecting me to lay out a simple prescription for what to do and the biochemical basis for it. What I see holding most people back from an optimized life is not a lack of information on how to eat and exercise, but a lack of buy-in, motivation, engagement, or discipline in honing particular areas of life. You must first focus on priming your mind before you will follow through with a life habit of optimizing your complex and nuanced machine. Your mindset, perspective, and attitude drive development in these areas. I hope to hereby pique your interest and curiosity about how you are designed to function, and help you identify areas ripe for growth.

Each heading below suggests a different construct that should make you consider how your machine is running, with improvements that can be implemented in and of themselves. I expand briefly on select constructs, and if you wish to dig deeper (which I wholeheartedly encourage), volumes have been written about each for your further investigation. Here, the goal is more modest: for you to see how a few basic and higher-level components interrelate. Although I separate the concepts to help you analyze yourself from different angles, remember that these parts work synergistically: the result of them coming together is far greater than the sum of the parts. Optimizing and integrating these facets of your design will lead you towards the life you were meant to live, with the freedom and function that we were all designed to enjoy. I hope you enjoy the perpetual journey of getting to know the systems comprising the amazing machine that is you.

Obstacles and Adversity: Bring It On!

It seems natural to try and avoid pain, but we grow only outside our comfort zones. Adversity is the breeding ground for the better you. Coaches manufacture it. Colleges look for it. Some even contend that God Himself provides for it. But we tend to dodge it. Our bodies, minds, and spirits are all designed to grow and get stronger by encountering and overcoming challenges. Yet most of our society teaches us to avoid challenges and lead lives of leisure, devoid of the trials and tribulations that provide the greatest potential to make us healthy and whole.

Rather than avoiding challenges, embrace them. This is often understood in the context of physical challenge—in a gym, surfing, mountain climbing, or similar activities—but the same lessons apply to our daily lives. In order to really stimulate our bodies to adapt and overcome, we need to reframe the obstacles encountered in our daily lives as opportunities. In other arenas, such as physical fitness, where the obstacles may not seem to stalk us as they do elsewhere, we need to actively seek out higher mountains to climb, new adventures to conquer, and the like. Growth can take place through the challenges that find us as well as those we pursue - if we have the positive mindset to attack them as the opportunities for growth that they are.

Nutrition: Fuel the Machine for the Journey

We were built as a hunter/gatherer. Our biology has not changed even as society and people's opinion of what's "normal" has. No one climbed a tree looking for fruit and came down with a cheesecake. Like gasoline in a race car, the quality and quantity of the fuel we put in the machine will greatly affect our performance. Junk food is not the high-octane (nutrition) we were designed to run on. This requires attention and discipline. Race teams do not carry extra gas cans in the backseat, nor do they water down race fuel. Neither should we. The hunter/gatherer in us generally survived on a plant-based diet, with some meat thrown in there when the hunt was good. But added sugars and processed foods were as foreign to them as they are ubiquitous today. So, seek those colorful natural foods that operate within you as high-performance fuels, and adopt the intentionality of fueling your body healthfully.

Exercise: Use It or Lose It

A car, left in a garage for decades, will no longer run. You are infinitely more complex than any car, but like a car, you are designed for constant use, not stagnation. Just like gravity, atrophy is an inescapable law of science. Your body (as well as your mind and spirit) need to be exercised in order to stay healthy. Remember the hunter/gatherer that you were designed to be? If a hunter/gatherer did not exercise, they did not eat!

Proper attention to your cardiovascular fitness, strength, and flexibility will keep your body optimized, just as proper training and "exercise" of your mind and spirit will ward off atrophy in those arguably even more critical areas. Depending on your age and present condition, your goals will vastly differ. I'm not insisting everyone sign up for the next marathon—a consistent walking program is a great routine for most (and, not coincidentally, probably what that hunter/gatherer did most). However, wherever you are, level up your daily routine in order to fend off the negative, stiffening effects caused by disuse.

Sleep: The Most Potent and Neglected Recovery Tool

I know I am not alone in my ongoing search for the 28-hour day, but my attempts to wean myself off sleep in the name of productivity have long been thwarted. Increasingly, science demonstrates that our human mechanism is utterly dependent on sleep, whether we fully understand why or not. From mental and physical performance, physical healing and recovery, and quality of life metrics, we learn that more is hampered or helped by sleep than we believe.

Even though sacrificing "productive" hours in the name of sleep may be the toughest thing for a driven person to do, you must make developing a good sleep rhythm a priority and seek help if necessary. While we all have somewhat differing needs, evidence suggests that most people do best averaging between seven and nine hours of sleep nightly. Again, I refer you to your hunter/gatherer self: your routine was fairly consistent every day. You woke up with the sun (to exercise) and did not have electronic screens keeping you up late into the night. Go and do likewise.

Stress Management: Keep the Needle in an Optimal Range

The word "stress" is overused and needs a more neutral definition. Certainly, stress can be very negative with too much stress leaving a person feeling depressed, suffocated, lacking energy, sleepless, or hopeless. Finding tools to help in those situations are critical. But some degree of "stress" is positive and probably what we were designed for—to bend but not break us.

Not only can the human body handle stress, it needs it. Muscles and bones, the brain and spirit all grow because of stress. Through micro-traumas we may not even detect, beautifully complex biochemical signals help regenerative pathways and develop synapse connections so that through stress, we grow, both psychologically and spiritually. To categorically avoid stress is a terrible goal. However, moderating and managing the dose, the timing, the preparation for, and the types of stress—these will determine whether the stimulus breaks you down or builds you up. When you look for the regeneration and growth that comes from an appropriate amount of stress, you will see that appropriate stress can be your friend rather than just a foe.

Rest, Rejuvenation, Relaxation, and Recreation: Make It Intentional

Rest is not just the absence of work or exertion, and properly defined, it is not only a passive process. "Rest" can be physically challenging and even exhausting yet rejuvenating for the soul. Rest may exercise parts of your brain that do not get enough bandwidth most days. Reframe the concept of "rest" as an active process to recharge the batteries and reinvigorate the spirit and body. This will often yield better efficiency in the long run, allowing you to fire on all cylinders when you are balanced and rejuvenated going back to "work". I am reminded that in scripture, even God took a day off—probably so He could rest up to deal with us afterwards. It is amusing to think that we do not recognize our need to do likewise.

Just like sleep, rest can be difficult to prioritize for "high performers." Ask yourself what type of rest and relaxation best recharges or rejuvenates you. Stopping and giving yourself time and space to just be calm certainly has a role and needs to be given permission and even priority. But potent rejuvenation can also come in many forms that we often do not consider—from meditation to exercise, from art to reading to volunteering—so explore what these and other forms of recharging your batteries on a regular basis might look like… and think about it on a contemplative walk this evening, for starters.

Operation Optimism: Who's Flying This Thing, Anyway?

Most machines have no attitude; they perform as built. However, as you well know, that's not us. The human machine has tremendous potential to operate as an overcomer or a victim. The optimism or pessimism you put in the driver's seat of this magnificent machine is what connects the lower, more base levels of mechanical function (physical health, etc.,) to the higher, more sophisticated levels of human function (relationships, generosity, grace) that we were designed for. A victorious spirit or an atrophic soul? Learn to thrive in the half-full part of the glass until it overflows; drive out darkness with light. Both your mental outlook and your physical health will benefit from focusing on the positive and the potential rather than the inevitable gaps and areas of lack in your life.

Faith: The Forgotten Factor and Possible Superpower

This may be the most difficult factor to analogize to a "machine" because humans have yet to fathom a machine so intricate as to approach having a soul or faith. But societies throughout human history have been driven by a universal quest for connection to a higher power, testifying to a spiritual nature that pleads for our attention. But the vast majority of us are too preoccupied, too uncomfortable discussing it, or too superficial to notice. And in doing so, we lose the potential of what may be our deepest purpose, connection, and drive. So, do not let this superpower lie unused. Spending time exploring and even wrestling with difficult questions of your faith or spirituality can bring fresh perspective to life in ways that little else can. Although expressed in a variety of ways, cultures throughout the world testify to elements of energy, health, peace, belonging, love, and freedom that can come from being actively engaged with faith—despite the fact that so many of us live in cultures that so easily drown it out.

Generosity and Gratitude: Reflecting How It All Comes Together

While diet and exercise (fuel and movement) are more basic levels of the machinery of our body, I would group generosity (along with gratitude, forgiveness, appreciation of beauty, and the like) as higher order operations that provide invaluable insight as to how well we are truly working. Generosity as a character trait, for example, requires far more than the basics required for self-sufficiency. It incorporates compassion and optimism with a perspective on our interrelatedness and trust in the future. It is a multifaceted output that demonstrates that many elements of the machine are doing well. Look for ways to be generous and develop a mindset of generosity in thought and deed. You will like yourself more and inspire others to do the same.

Forgiveness, Grace, and Humility: High-Level Signs of Health and Repairing

We all do things that we should not. We all fall short of our potential. We eat and drink too much or the wrong things; we exercise too little or too much or in ways we should not; we damage long-term relationships, trust, and genuine love through short-sighted selfishness and petty gain. It is called being human. Volumes, religions, and entire philosophies of living have developed around guiding people through these frustrating inevitabilities of the human condition. Fortunately, most sophisticated machines are designed with the anticipation that certain parts will break and wear out. We are no exception, but reparations do not come easily. To not learn from our experiences would be foolish, however holding grudges or resentment towards others is more likely to hurt us than the other person, both mentally and physically. Our bodies don't do well while harboring unhealthy feelings towards others – or towards ourselves. This chapter in the "owner's manual" needs to be studied and practiced repeatedly for the higher-level functions of grace, humility, and forgiveness to really become a habit. In doing so, we can often keep our, and others' inevitable "failures" from turning into catastrophic or terminal ones.

Goals: We Go and Grow Nowhere Without Them

We were not meant to simply exist, adrift and blown by the wind and the current. Such a fate leaves us shipwrecked and squanders all we were made for. We were meant to have meaning and purpose in many areas of our lives. Bookstores are filled with great exhortation and inspiration to make our goals more achievable, well defined, and fulfilling. From pondering the "why" behind these goals, to developing the accountability and discipline to achieve them, you may discover that you were meant for more than you have ever imagined. So, start setting goals. Set goals for your body, your mind, and your spirit. Setting goals is one of the surest ways to wake up excited about growing into who you want to become. No matter where you are in your level of fitness, eating habits, and overall mindset, you have the ability to change. Some old dogs do learn new tricks—but not the ones who do not try. You may need to start with baby steps, but every marathoner started that way. The one strategy that will not get your there is postponement. A better you is waiting just around the corner.

Final Words

I started by describing the importance of critically analyzing how we were designed and evolved to function optimally. I touched on nutrition, exercise, sleep habits, stress management, and relaxation as some basic but critical components for developing and maintaining a successful body. Now ask yourself what changes you could make in these areas that would get your body closer to the machine it is capable of becoming.

I also highlighted some ways that higher-level programming of our body manifests, including optimism, faith, generosity, forgiveness, and gratitude. Spend some introspective time being curious as to which of these areas needs most development, and even asking why. Set small goals and start building the habit of achieving them. We all have areas in which we could improve, but therein lies the opportunity for a better you—not an excuse for complacency. Just as with nutrition and exercise, set goals and imagine the potential you that is out there. The degree of introspection, research, and goal setting you apply to your own mind and body will have dramatic implications on the areas in which you grow, stagnate, or fall apart. Success is an ongoing journey as you change over the years—but the approach, analysis, and growth can be continuous—and I wish you Godspeed for the journey.

About the Author

Dave Wallis is a family and sports medicine physician in Hermosa Beach, California. He is a five-time Ironman finisher and has completed the Boston Marathon, Paris-Brest-Paris, many other triathlons, and a variety of other crazy events in his perpetual endeavor to create great memories and live life to its fullest. He has close to 20 years' experience working with professional athletes and sports teams including US Soccer, the LA Galaxy, Chivas USA, and the Los Angeles Dodgers. He has authored over a dozen medical publications and currently does public speaking, pharmaceutical consulting, and has a small concierge medicine practice. He has been blessed to travel the world and loves learning from the beauty of cultures all over. But his greatest gifts, pride, and joy are his four kids and his amazing wife—who has loved him well and put up with him for decades.

Email: doctorwallis@yahoo.com

CHAPTER 33

A BIBLICAL PERSPECTIVE ON LIVING LIKE AN OLYMPIC CHAMPION

By Dr. Dave White, PhD
NCAA Men's Basketball Referee, Success Life Coach and Mentor
Los Angeles, California

No one understood the "successful body" better than the ancient Greeks. No historical event better captures the "successful body" than the ancient Olympic Games, founded 28 centuries ago in 776 BC. Apart from giving us philosophy, geometry, drama, art, and science, you can thank the ancient Greeks for our inordinate passion for youth, the body, physical culture, and sports. The blood and guts, sinew and muscle that marked the Olympic contests is unmatched in time.

But this "festival of physicality" was much more than just sport. It was seen as the showcase of heart and harmony, virtue and valor, soul, integrity, wholeness, and manhood. Olympia was seen as the meeting place of heaven and earth—layered with religious ceremonies, music concerts, and the ultimate entertainment package. Picture the modern Olympic Games combined with the Carnival in Rio, a week at the Magic Kingdom and Easter Mass at the Vatican. For five hectic days and nights, Olympia was the place to be.

The second century satirist, Lucian, wrote this, about his experience:

> If the Olympic Games were being held right now, you would see why we Greeks attach such paramount importance to athletics. Oh, I can't describe the scene in mere words. You really should experience firsthand the incredible pleasure of standing in that cheering crowd, admiring the athletes' courage and good looks, their amazing physical conditioning—their great skill and irresistible strength—all their bravery and their pride, their unbeatable determination, their unstoppable passion for victory! I know if you were there in the Stadium, you wouldn't be able to stop applauding. (Lucian, Anacharsis, CAD 140)

As Lucian stated, the Olympic Games not only showcased good-looking, conditioned, skilled, strong successful bodies, they highlighted inspiring human courage, bravery, determination, and passion. Given this, it's no wonder that many writers such as Homer, Lucian, Herodotus, Thucydides, and Pausanias used sports in their works.

Even the Biblical writers used Olympic imagery to describe portions of the Christian life because they were such revered and celebrated symbols of the ancient world. New Testament writers such as Luke, the Apostle Paul, and the writer of Hebrews all used athletic metaphors.

The Olympic Games were a big deal. Dean Stanley notes that the games were to the Greeks, what the temple was to the Jews and what the triumph was to the Romans. Greek citizens could visualize the games like Americans can visualize Pearl Harbor, the assassination of President Kennedy, the Space Shuttle Challenger explosion, or the 9/11 attacks.

Ancients had a "mental map" of the games. They could visualize the Olympic venues and events—along with the pathway to the prize. Biblical writers assume we too have this "mental map" and can use this knowledge as a bridge to exhort us to live the life of a heroic champion.

Let me help you visualize this too. Join me at eight historic Olympic venues. Each of these venues points to a core championship value. And each value is mentioned in the Bible to inspire us to reach our best selves beyond just the physical. Here's a simple chart listing the **venues** with their **values** and **verses**.

Venues	Values	Variations	Verses
1. The Gym	Train Hard	Physically	(1 Timothy 4:7–8)
2. The Temple	Compete Honorably	Spiritually	(2 Timothy 2:5)
3. The Stripping Room	Strip Down	Emotionally	(Hebrews 12:1)
4. The Stadium	Run Your Race	Relationally	(Hebrews 12:1)
5. The Track	Run to Win	Mentally	(1 Corinthians 9:24–27)
6. The Pole	Run with Aim	Volitionally	(Hebrews 12:2-3; Philippians 3)
7. The Finish Line	Finish Strong	Personally	(Acts 20:24; 2 Timothy 4:7–8)
8. The Bema Seat	Inspire Others	Socially	(Philippians 2:16; 1 Cor. 3:10–15)

Want both a "successful body" and a "successful being?" Desire a "successful physique" and also a "successful faith?" Eager to live the life of a heroic Olympic champion with a perfected body and polished mentality? If so, then journey with me to Olympia. First stop, the gymnasium.

Venue 1: The Gym
Value: Train Hard (Physically)
As an Olympian trains with specialized coaches to discipline their body physically, be diligent to stay healthy and fit. Work out hard, feed your frame good nutrition, stay hydrated, and get ample sleep. In addition, find mentors and coaches to help you to develop your fitness, hobbies, platform, and business. Most importantly, work with the best, to be the best, in your heart, soul, and mind.

Verse: 1 Timothy 4:8. *Train yourself to be godly. For physical training is of some value, but godliness has value for all things. It holds promise for both the present life and the future life to come.*

The Greek word "gymnazo," from which we get our English word "gymnasium," refers to the kind of training and working out that takes place in a serious gym and athletic training center. Champions prepared and practiced, disciplined and drilled, exercised and exerted themselves. They pushed, pulled, and pumped their way to exceptional fitness. They submitted to regimented routines and systematic stress to condition themselves for peak performance.

The apostle Paul exhorts us all to do that, not just to be great physical specimens, but to be great spiritual beings—good, honest, ethical, virtuous, noble, principled, wholesome, and reverent people.

He argues that while physical training, bodily discipline, fitness, and exercise ("somatiky gymnasia"), have some benefit and profit, somatic strength is limited. The payoff of a great core, constitution, and carriage is modest, in extent and duration, compared with having great character.

Being in good shape physically feels great but is temporary and transient. Being in good shape spiritually is timeless and transcendent. The benefits are powerful and permanent, extensive and eternal.

Venue 2: The Temple
Value: Compete Honorably (Spiritually)

As an Olympian makes a sacred oath to compete ethically, according to the rules of the game, do your part to live an ethically and spiritually rich life. Character matters. If you're a person of faith, build your life consistent with God's rulebook (the Bible) and a strong ethical code you can be proud of.

Verse: 2 Timothy 2:5. *If anyone competes or contends as an athlete, he does not win or receive the prize unless he competes according to the RULES.*

The Apostle Paul reminds his young disciple Timothy that if anyone wants to participate as an "athleo," they better be courageous. Like the ancient hoplite soldier, the athletic grappler, wrestler, boxer, and runner were competitive contenders. Athletes are fighters—fighting fatigue, fighting the flesh, and fighting their own finitude with healthy bodies, strong minds, and robust wills.

Olympians were classy contenders. They had an ethic about them. These were not the brutish, beastly gladiator contests in Rome. These were not savage spectacles of antiquity. The Olympics were top-notch games. Champions played by the rules—lawfully and fairly. You cannot win the victor's crown, the champion's wreath, or the gold medal by cutting corners, cheating, or playing illegally.

Venue 3: The Stripping Room
Value: Strip Down (Emotionally)

As an Olympian strips their body to compete, lean, mean, and unencumbered, they also do so to rid themselves of any emotional unresolved baggage that could slow them down. Courage and candor were needed to compete nude. Less is more. While it is healthy to strip our bodies of excess weight, we should also be ripped emotionally. Do your part to eliminate any unresolved hurts, hang-ups, and habits that could bog you down in the race. Shed dead weight in your schedule, excess in your relationships, and unsavory behaviors in your life that slow you down from reaching your goals.

Verse: Hebrews 12:1–2. *Throw off everything that hinders and the sin that so easily entangles.*

The "apo-dyterion" was the ancient changing room in Roman bath houses, where warrior-athletes disrobed from their chitons (light tunics) and got "gym-nos," meaning "naked," so they could scrape and shave their bodies with the strigil. Man-scaped contenders were primarily concerned with eliminating all that hindered to win their contests. But Greek and Roman competitors acknowledge they also primped and preened with oils and powders to look healthy, glistening, and inspiring to their followers.

Running in a long, ancient toga is a great illustration of a disaster. As you can imagine, a sprinter would easily be constricted, slowed down, and tripped up running in the equivalent of a bathrobe. Off with everything. Anything that diverts our attention, saps our energy, dampens our enthusiasm, or handicaps our journey should be jettisoned.

To stay emotionally healthy, say goodbye to unmanageable schedules, unredeemed weekends, unfortunate debt, unhealthy relationships, unresolved conflicts, unnecessary guilt, and unprocessed emotional baggage. Busy calendars, over-extended commitments, and a frantic lifestyle need to go too.

Venue 4: The Stadium
Value: Run Your Race (Relationally)

As an Olympian runs with endurance cheered on by their fans, don't try to achieve your most demanding goals by yourself. Ancient athletes had faithful followers, a relational tribe of fans who quickened them to be their best. For epic results, marshal meaningful relationships around you. Have a coach.

Build good friends. Develop a support system to surround you. And remember who you are—your identity ties you to your family history and your spiritual heritage as an additional incentive to continue in the race.

Verse: Hebrews 12:1. *As believers, since we, ourselves, are surrounded by such a great cloud of witnesses, let us run with perseverance the race marked out for us.*

Because we are relationally encompassed by a huge host of amazing martyrs (Greek word "marturon"), we should run accordingly. Generations of amazing men and women have finished strong before us. They did it. We can do it. The metaphorical use of a "cloud" was a common classical way to describe something incredible and massive. (Homer, Herodotus, and Virgil used it.) Imagine an encircling amphitheater, with its ascending row upon row of enthusiastic spectators. Our historical heritage is awesome! We run motivated relationally to join their ranks.

Athletes are called to trek (from the Greek word "trek-omen") with "perseverance"—for the race before them was an "agona" (Greek for "agony"). Champions will need determination to overcome the inevitable discouragements along the long marathon. The contest can be crushing. The journey is difficult and demanding, exhausting and excruciating, tiring, taxing, and torturous.

The race is arduous for us all. But know this—you have what it takes. The grueling contest you face has been personally prescribed for you. It's a uniquely marked-out quest. The individual road you are called to travel has been specially set before you by God Himself. So, don't copy others. And don't rebuff the course He has set you on. Run your race!

Venue 5: The Track:
Value: Run to Win (Mentally)

As an Olympian takes the track with a winning mindset and runs all-out to win Olympic glory, live your life intentionally with a champions' mentality. Cerebral strength matters. A brawny brain makes a difference. Do all you can to develop a fortified mind—thoughtful, long-suffering, able to delay gratification, and unregulated by externals. Your alpha attitudes and actions will be immensely practical in your day-to-day life but will be particularly rewarding in the eternal state.

Verse: 1 Corinthians 9:24–27. *Do you not know that in a race all the athletic runners run, but only one gets the prize, run in such a way that you may win. Everyone who competes in the games exercises self-control in all things. They go into strict training. They do it to receive a perishable wreath but we an imperishable. Therefore I run in such a way, as not without aim; I box in such a way, as not beating the air; but I discipline my body and make it my slave, so that, after I have preached to others I myself will not be disqualified.*

Paul uses Olympic language to exhort us. He wants us to win. Of course, winning was a life-and-death issue in the ancient world. Countries with the best athletes had the best armies. There is no second place in war. It's win and live, or lose and die.

This mentality is foreign to most moderners. Today many value passivity and participation, not aggressiveness and competition. Moderners value effort, not success, doing one's personal best, not winning. The modern Olympic Creed reflects this, saying, "The most important thing in the Olympic Games is <u>not to win</u> but to <u>take part</u>, just as the most important thing in life is <u>not the triumph</u> but the struggle. The essential thing is <u>not to have conquered</u> but to have fought well."

Not win, not triumph, not conquer. Simply to take part, to struggle, and to have fought well? To Biblical writers, this wouldn't make sense at all. Our forefathers were fierce champion-warriors who valued not only participation but a mentality of winning.

Venue 6: The Pole
Value: Run with Aim (Volitionally)

As an Olympian runs undistracted and focused on the finish line pole, choose to be strategically riveted. Having the end in mind allows you to make sure every step zeroes in on your goal. Knowing your health and nutrition goals is important. And so is knowing your lane in life, avoiding comparing yourself with others, and centering your attention on your targeted aims.

Verse: Hebrews 12:2. *Let us fix our eyes on Jesus, the author and perfecter of our faith.*

The writer highlights the finish line pole, so contenders feel strengthened and encouraged to continue on, with a hopeful horizon to aim for. Believers were to courageously fixate on the personal, human, relatable Jesus who Himself endured pain and suffering. Look locked on the Lord. Not looking around. Not distracted. Not side-tracked. The Greek word "aphorao" is used here; it means to look away from all else and to fix one's gaze exclusively on the goal. As the Apostle Paul told the Philippians, "I press on toward the goal for the prize" (Philippians 3:14). He strained and stretched every nerve and muscle with ceaseless exertion and intense desire to win the race and to receive the prize.

Venue 7: The Finish Line
Value: Finish Strong (Personally)
As an Olympian endures the marathon to the very end, do everything you can to finish strong. Marathoners are a rare breed—a very select group of warriors. Ironmen have personal prowess, grit, and gravitas unmatched by most. In life, see the big picture, strategize for the long game. Keep yourself healthy, continue to refine your aligned destiny, pace yourself where needed, and go the distance in completing your calling.

Verse: Acts 20:24. *I consider my life worth nothing to me, if only I may finish the race and complete the task the Lord Jesus has given me—the task of testifying to the gospel of God's grace.*

What's your calling in life? What's your ultimate goal? What legacy do you want to leave? Here Luke records for us Paul's closing sentiments at the end of his life. The apostle wanted to finish the race doing exactly what God personally called him to do—sharing, proclaiming, and advocating for the good news, namely the gospel of God's amazing grace.

Venue 8: The Bema Seat
Value: Inspire Others (Socially)
As an Olympian competes to win the crown, prestige, and glory of a victor, do your work with excellence, conduct your relationships with the highest attention to detail, and live your life intentionally for the things that truly last. As athletic champions inspire others with their feats, use your accomplishments to build a social platform where you can inspire and serve others. Use your expertise as an opportunity to bless others and to bring value to the world.

Verse: Philippians 2:16. *I did not run or labor for nothing.*

In the ancient Olympic Games, victors were honored with a montage of benefits from spectator applause, to being crowned with a wreath of olive, parsley, laurel, or pine by the Hellanodikaia on a raised platform. The pomp and pageantry included triumphal processions, an official parade, sacrifices to thank the gods, banquets with compatriots, a plaque on the city gate, and even exemption from the military and from taxes. Special songs, poems, and benefits continued throughout the victors' lives. Special honored seats at social and stately events were often given. Many times, they were honored with a statue of themselves for all to see.

Paul uses this knowledge to remind people of faith that eternal awards await their efforts. Paul did not marathon like an Olympic runner in ministry for no good. His work and toil were not useless or in vain. A reward remained.

In Conclusion

As I shared before, no one understood the "successful body" better than the ancient Greeks. No historical event better captures the "successful body" than the ancient Olympic Games. Even the Biblical writers used Olympic imagery to describe portions of the Christian life because they were such revered and celebrated symbols of the ancient world.

Ancients had a "mental map" of the games. They could visualize the Olympic venues and events—along with the pathway to the prize. Biblical writers assume we too have that "mental map" and can use that knowledge as a bridge to exhort us to live the life of a heroic champion.

Want both a "successful body" and a "successful being?" Desire a "successful physique" and also a "successful faith?" Want to live an Olympic heroic life? Then use the eight Olympic venues to remind you of eight Olympic values (supported by eight Biblical verses) to living a heroic championship life.

By remembering the eight elements below and taking action to mirror these ancient suggestions, you can continually build upon your successful body, successful mind, and successful spirit to reach a lofty goal, just as the ancient Olympic champions did.

1. The Gym reminds you to Train Hard (Physically).
2. The Temple reminds you to Compete Honorably (Spiritually).
3. The Stripping Room reminds you to Strip Down (Emotionally).
4. The Stadium reminds you to Run Your Race (Relationally).

5. The Track reminds you to Run to Win (Mentally).
6. The Pole reminds you to Run with Aim (Volitionally).
7. The Finish Line reminds you to Finish Strong (Personally).
8. The Bema Seat reminds you to Inspire Others (Socially).

About the Author

On the court, Dr. Dave White is a lead NCAA Men's basketball referee. He's known for controlling the game, making big calls under pressure, and managing passionate alpha coaches and intense competitive players.

Off the court, Dave is a men's business success life coach for athletes, executives, entrepreneurs, and workplace warriors. He champions champions and influences influencers, so they can get control of their game, make important calls, manage the pressure, and seize the winning results they want.

Dave is a UCLA grad with a PhD in Education. He's traveled to 70 countries and lived in four of them. He's passionate about the Olympic movement, staying in shape, and serving God. He's happily married to his wife Sue of 34 years. Together they have five grown children, two sons-in-law, a daughter-in-law, and a beautiful granddaughter.

Email: dave@drdavewhite.com
Website: www.drdavewhite.com

CHAPTER 34

SEVEN HABITS TO CHANGE YOUR LIFE

By Erik Seversen
Author, Speaker, Coach
Los Angeles, California

I have a confession to make. I'm not a health expert. I'm not a personal trainer, and I don't know the science of nutrition. Indeed, there are many people who know a lot more than I do about fitness, nutrition, and mindset, which is exactly why I chose to reach out to the experts to help me create this book, *The Successful Body*.

Now that the book is finished, as I read the chapters, I'm glad (and I'm sure you are too) that I didn't try to complete this task alone. Rather, I found personal trainers, nutritionists, and mindset experts who could help you with your health goals. But, in the end, as I learned more about the body while reaching out to health and well-being professionals to help co-author this book, I realized that fitness, nutrition, and mindset are only parts of the puzzle that make up a healthy body. I learned about factors that might damage the body, including corporate stress, chronic inflammation, environmental toxicity, food addiction, physical injury, sleep deprivation, and other deleterious lifestyle habits. I also learned about some techniques to combat these issues, for example, eating real foods, meditating, using mental toughness, boxing, setting goals, transforming from the inside out, detoxifying your body, using strength training, overcoming harmful emotions, and simply moving to stay healthy. I learned how all of these are part of a universe of factors that determine a person's health, success, and happiness.

No, I'm not a human body expert, but I'm happy to say that currently, in my 50th year on earth, I'm in good shape. At 50, I ran a marathon (finishing with nearly the same time I did 15 years earlier); I climbed Mt. Elbrus, the 18,510-foot peak in the Caucasus Mountain range in southern Russia marking the highest point in Europe; I rode a motorcycle thousands of miles through the mountains and deserts of Morocco; weekly, I surfed with my kids; and generally, I've felt healthy, energetic, and alive. I wouldn't call my levels of fitness and health "extreme," and I didn't do anything radical to get my body into shape; rather, I simply decided to copy the positive habits of some other successful people. And this, I think, is what allows me to live an active life, free from limiting physical boundaries.

I hope you've already made some life-style changes based on the content from this book, and I'm going to leave you now with just a few things that, for me, are foundational to the physical and mental state that allows me the freedom to do the things I love. Basically, these are very simple, almost too simple, habits that have dramatically improved my life.

My personal journey to a stronger mind and body started when I created a company in 2016. I was still working in a corporate job doing international business development, and I knew that I needed to make some changes to get the edge I needed to essentially put energy into two jobs and a family. I began by studying mostly business and inspirational giants such as Tim Ferriss, Tony Robbins, Brendon Burchard, and others. This led me to see some of the habits of uber-successful people. I realized that thought leaders, top-performing professional athletes, billionaires, and other successful people seemed to share a distinct set of habits. Below are some of the things I found most common among them. I didn't have to reinvent the wheel to create a body that allowed me the energy to reach my goals. All I had to do was copy the common habits of these people. Here, I'll outline seven simple habits that, if implemented, will change your life.

Habit 1—Breathe Deeply

Most humans simply don't breathe deeply enough. Shallow breaths are stealing our energy, especially if we spend much of the day sitting. To perform at an extraordinary level, we need as much oxygen flowing through our body as possible. You will feel immediate energy just after doing breathing exercises, and you will feel more focus during the day with this very simple act of breathing deeply.

All you have to do is *take three GIANT breaths, five times per day* (or more). Breathe in as deeply as you can, hold for 15 seconds, and release. Do this three times in a row, every two hours throughout the day. If you must, set a phone, clock, or e-calendar to remind you to take the breaths every two hours. Once you get into the habit of this, you'll find that you automatically take deep breaths whenever you need a quick boost of energy. It is like drinking a quick cup of coffee but without the jitters.

Habit 2—Drink Water

Like breathing, drinking water is simple, but very important. Although more people are proactive about staying hydrated, most people simply don't drink enough water. Our body functions much better with water. It is a life force within us, and, as with breathing deeply, you will feel immediate positive results in energy and focus with the simple act of drinking water.

All you have to do is *drink one full glass of water, five times per day.* There are two ways to do this. One is to drink a full glass of water every time you take your giant breaths every two hours (which is what I do). The other is to sip throughout the day, making sure you get five glasses.

Habit 3—Eat Quality Food

Poor eating habits are taking a giant toll on Americans as well as people all over the world. Certain types of diabetes and obesity are avoidable tragedies. Too much sugar, too much fat, and too many processed foods are making us sick and are slowing us down. Choose to be one of those who watches exactly what you put into your body as fuel. Eating right sounds simple enough, but we don't always add the best fuel to our bodies. Many people would benefit by radically modifying their eating habits for peak performance. At the start, a bit of common sense and tiny changes are all that is needed.

All you have to do to start is *snack mainly on fruits, add one extra portion of green vegetables to your daily meals, subtract sugary sodas, and consume moderate portions of food.* Just use common sense, with these three things in mind:

1. Green vegetables and all fruits are very good for you, so eat as many as you can.
2. Processed and packaged foods, and sugary sodas are not good for you, so consume them as seldomly as possible.
3. Moderate portions are better than eating too much.

Habit 4—Move Your Body

Exercise isn't just for athletes and gym enthusiasts. It is an extremely important key to high performance. When asked what the key to success is, Richard Branson is said to have simply answered, "Work out."

All you have to do to start is *30 minutes of cardio and five minutes of strength-building exercise, each day.* Base the exercise on your current fitness ability, but make sure you push yourself a bit.

The cardio part of the daily habit is a great time to include family. A walk, jog, or bike around the neighborhood after dinner is a great and feasible way to get in the cardio as well as bond with others. For the muscle-strengthening component, as with eating, just use common sense. It can be weights, kettlebells, bodyweight exercises, or whatever you want to do according to your equipment and ability. If you have no equipment for strength development, do bodyweight exercises, such as squats, sit-ups, push-ups, and arm curls (using a chair). I do this in four sets of 15 each, and it takes about five minutes. Again, do this to your fitness ability. Modify to knee push-ups and crunches if that is better for you. The main thing is to get into the habit of doing something. Also, the recommendation of 30 minutes and five minutes is to establish the routine but doing more is even better.

Habit 5—Meditate

This habit is fundamental to the routines of billionaires, sports icons, thought leaders, and pretty much all the peak performers in the world. This is a massively significant habit, and I think it is one of the most beneficial yet most neglected of all the recommended practices.

All you have to do is *dedicate 15 to 20 minutes every day to meditation.* Don't worry if your mind wanders; let your mind go wherever it wants to go. There is no right or wrong way to meditate, and there is no right or wrong time to meditate. Most of the people I know who meditate daily do it in the morning, but the methods vary significantly. Find the meditation that works best for you from sitting quietly for a duration of time, to using a vocally repeated mantra, to focused prayer, to following a guided meditation. Whatever you find, know that having a dedicated time to let your mind relax, flow, and simply exist is done by almost every single one of the world's highest achievers. Also, when I start to think that I'm too busy to take 15 minutes away from the start of my day, I remind myself that I'm consistently more productive throughout the day if I take the time to meditate, so the time spent reaps returns in dividends.

Habit 6—Prioritize

Working hard does not guarantee success. You need to make sure your efforts are spent on the things that produce results. This goes for school, business, and your health.

All you have to do is *track the progress of your health goals.* Frequently, make a list of the health goals you are working on and circle the most important things on that list. Then, decide what actions you must take to make progress in those areas. Tracking your progress helps keep things fun and helps keep you on track.

I think most people are aware of Pareto's Law or the 80/20 rule. This magical revelation by an Italian economist long ago has helped millions of people become more successful by helping them focus on what produces rather than what doesn't. In a nutshell, the 80/20 rule is that 20 percent of our efforts produce 80 percent of our results, so we need to discover which 20 percent of our work produces the highest output, and we need to spend more time on this rather than on the 80 percent effort that doesn't produce.

Habit 7—Celebrate

The ability to celebrate small and large successes is a great way to stay motivated. All you have to do is *remember to pause and celebrate when you reach daily, weekly, monthly, and yearly milestones.* The more you celebrate, the more excited you will be to continue, and the positive vibes you generate will not only benefit you but will be infectious to those around you.

Last Words

I know it can be daunting, sometimes, to filter through all the suggestions out there on how to be healthy. I hope this book has provided something that speaks to you. If you connected with anything particular in any of the chapters in this book, take action and decide to make a positive change right now. Contact any authors if you have further questions for them or if you'd like to get more personal help. No one can reach success totally on their own, but changing our bodies is within our control.

Ask yourself right now, "Am I happy with my body?" It really doesn't matter what anyone else thinks, but it does matter what you think. Evaluate the visual outline of your body, and, even more importantly, listen to your body and evaluate your internal health and well-being. Are you totally satisfied with where you are now, or are there some changes you would like to make? No matter where you are, from marathon-ready fit to overweight and sluggish, I pray that you challenge yourself to work toward and maintain the successful body you deserve. It is your body, and it is your choice whether your body works for or against you. Choose to have your body work for you, so you can feel better, look better, and reach your goals.

About the Author

Erik Seversen is on a mission to inspire people. He holds a master's degree in anthropology and is a certified practitioner of neuro linguistic programming. Erik draws from his years of teaching at the university level and years of real-life experience to motivate people to take action creating extreme success in business and in life.

Erik is an author of five books, keynote speaker, adventurer, entrepreneur, and educator who has traveled to 85 countries and all 50 states in the USA. His travels and intersections with people have been a deep study of love, struggle, and ways of thinking that Erik relies on to tackle challenges in school, business, and life. His most current ambitions are sharing the lessons he's learned with others and climbing mountains. Erik lives in Los Angeles with his wife and two boys.

This chapter, "Seven Habits to Change Your Life," is drawn from Erik's 24-page *Extraordinary Habits Challenge*. If you would like to download a free copy of the entire 21-day challenge outlining 10 success habits and 11 success behaviors, visit Erik's website. Also available on Erik's website are his other books, interviews, and writing resources for authors.

Email: Erik@ErikSeversen.com
Website: www.ErikSeversen.com

DID YOU ENJOY THIS BOOK?

If you enjoyed reading this book, you can help by suggesting it to someone else you think might like it, and **please leave a positive review** wherever you purchased it. This does a lot in helping others find the book. We thank you in advance for taking a few moments to do this.

THANK YOU

If you enjoyed reading this book, you might also like: ***The Successful Mind: Tools to Living a Purposeful, Productive, and Happy Life***

The Successful Mind is a co-authored book highlighting the importance of Mindset in reaching success. Since success isn't one thing, *The Successful Mind* was written by multiple authors from varying backgrounds, locations, and areas of expertise. The book is divided into three sections of Purpose, Productivity, and Happiness with author contributors writing stand-alone chapters that answer questions such as: What is the mindset required for success in business and entrepreneurship? How can meditation create a mindset of success? What is the mindset needed for positive change? Is there a mindset for economic success? What mindset can eliminate fear? Chapters include disciplines from science, humanities, business, sociology, and healthy living. The goal of the book is for authors to highlight their unique experiences regarding mindset and success, but for each message to be relatable to people from any walk of life.

Made in the USA
Columbia, SC
14 March 2021